Neurodegenerative Diseases - Molecular Mechanisms and Current Therapeutic Approaches

Edited by Nagehan Ersoy Tunalı

Published in London, United Kingdom

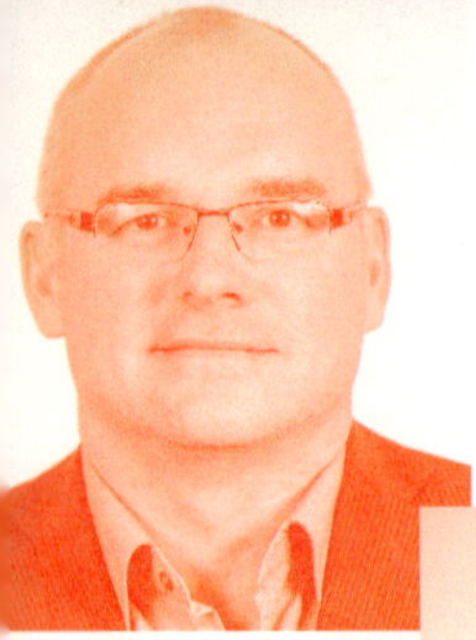
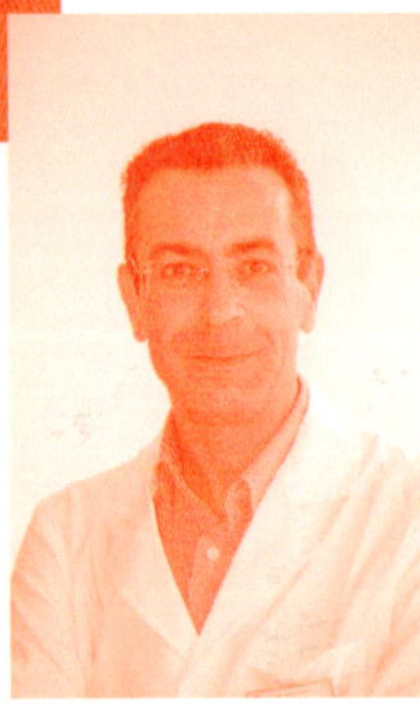
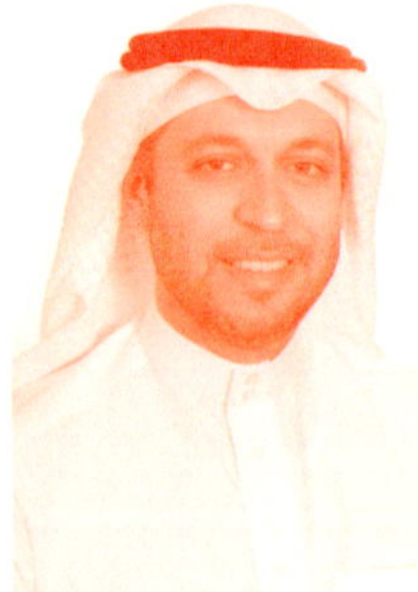
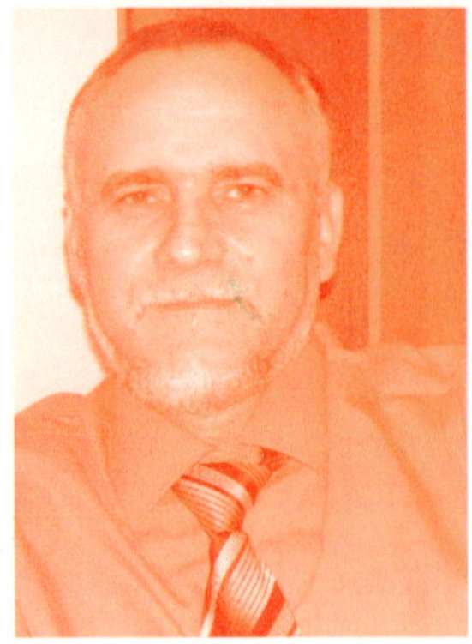
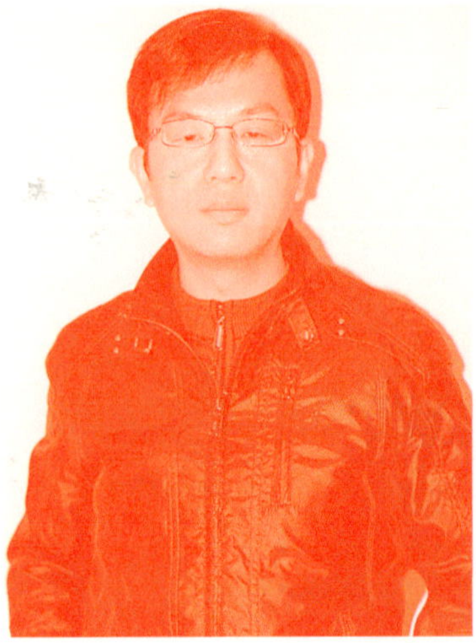
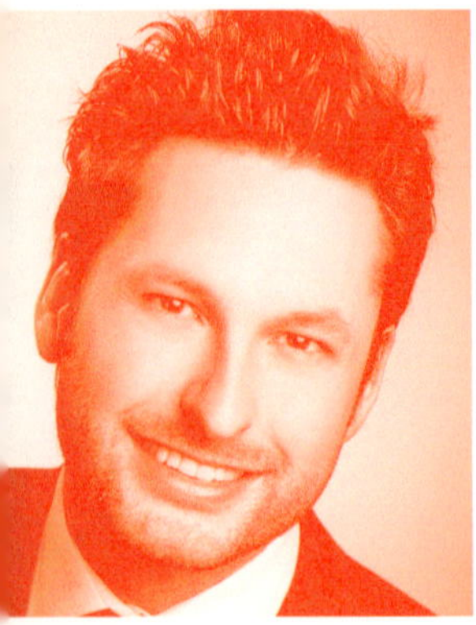
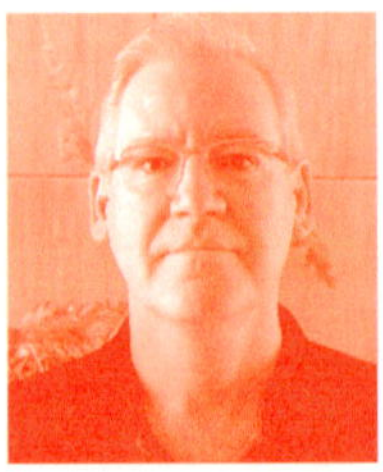

IntechOpen

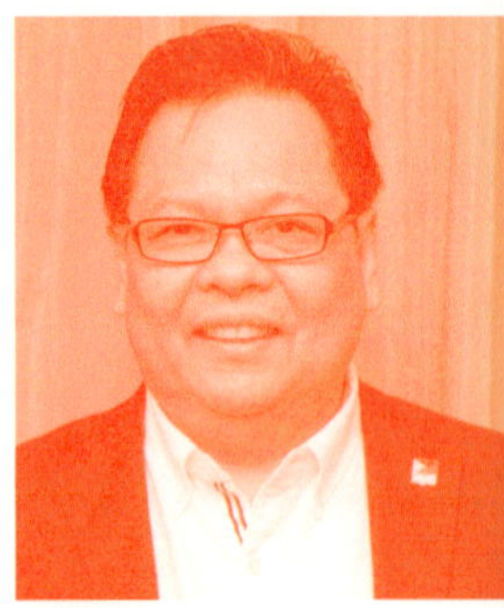
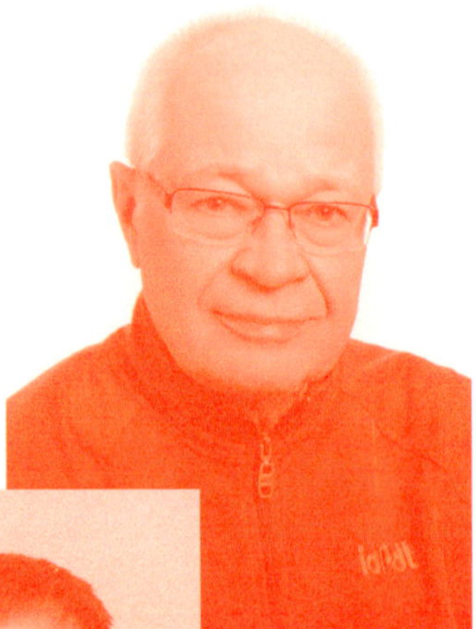
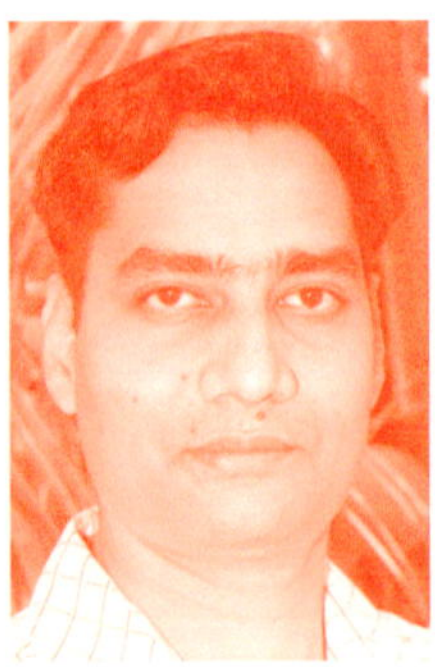
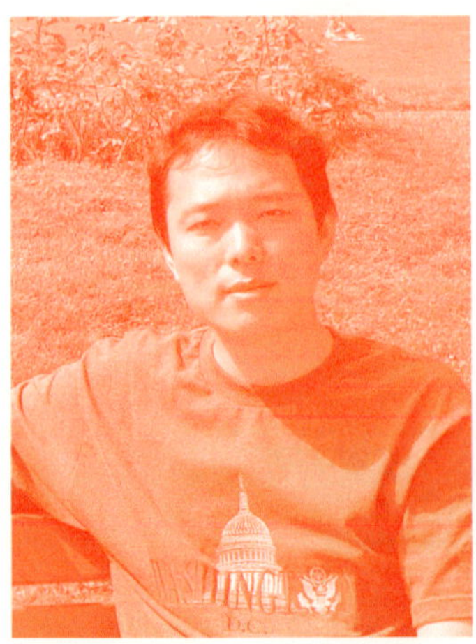
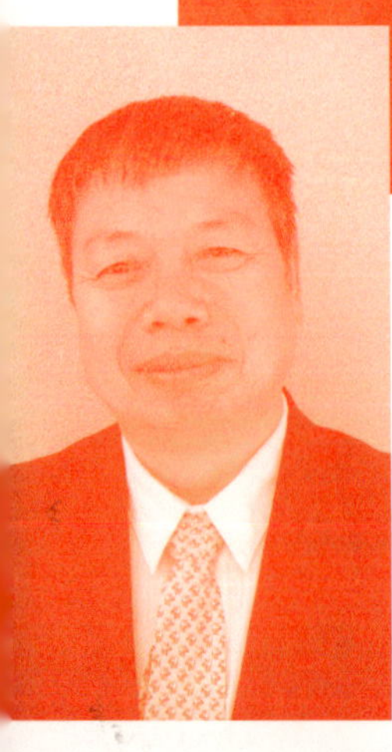
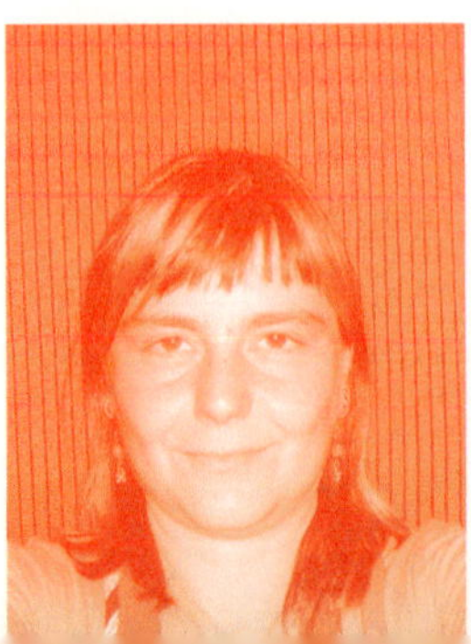

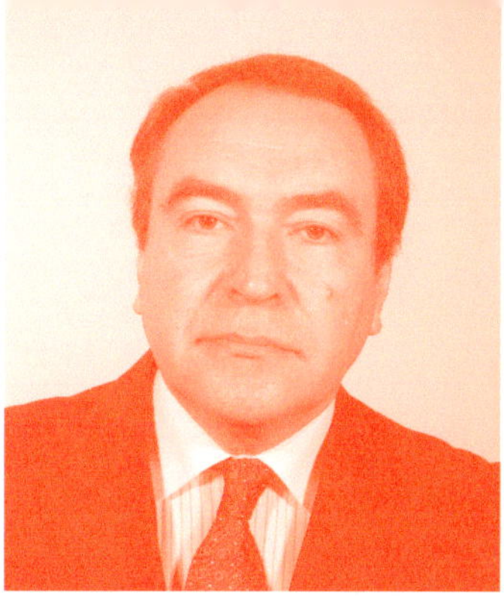
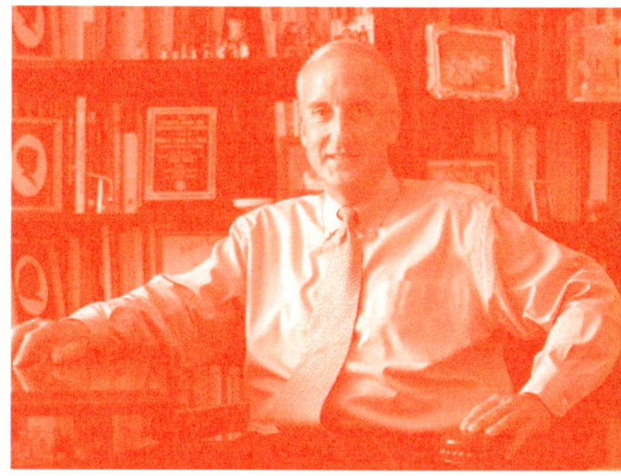
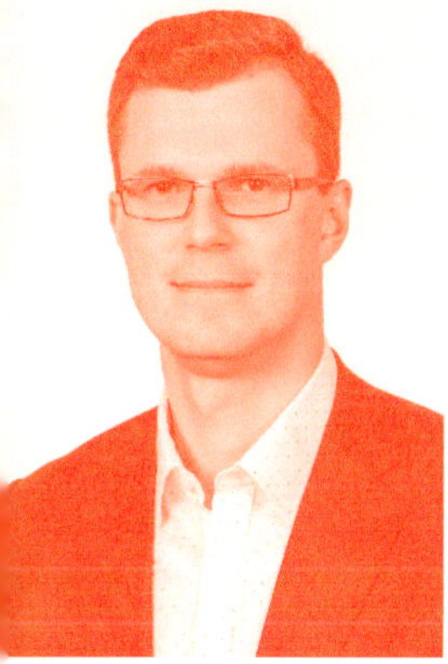
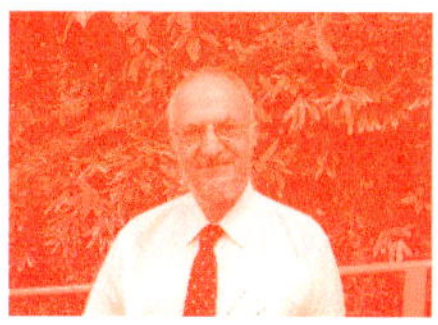
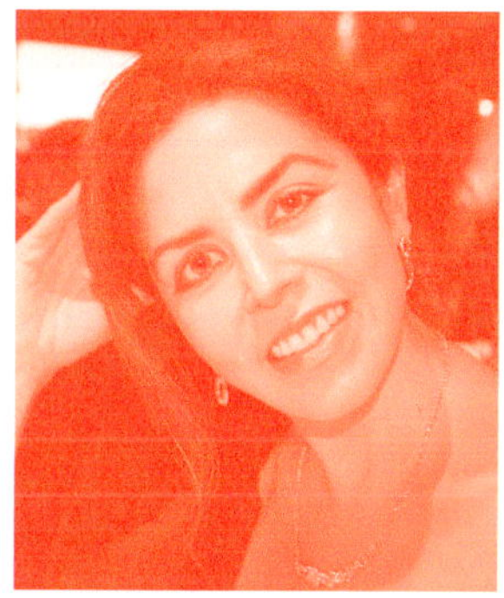

Supporting open minds since 2005

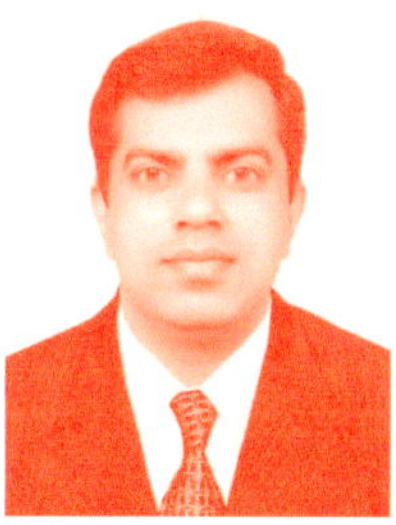
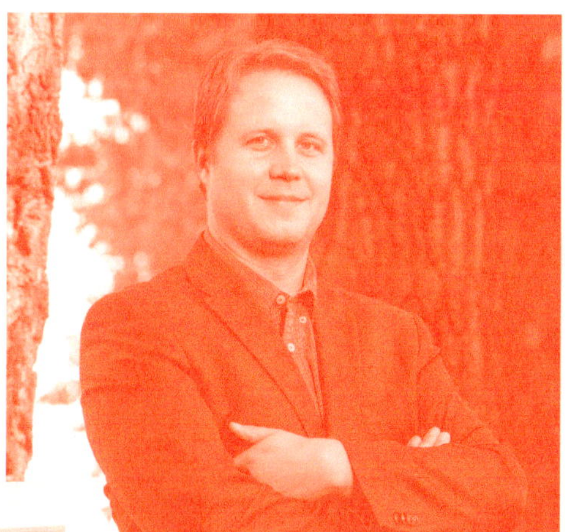
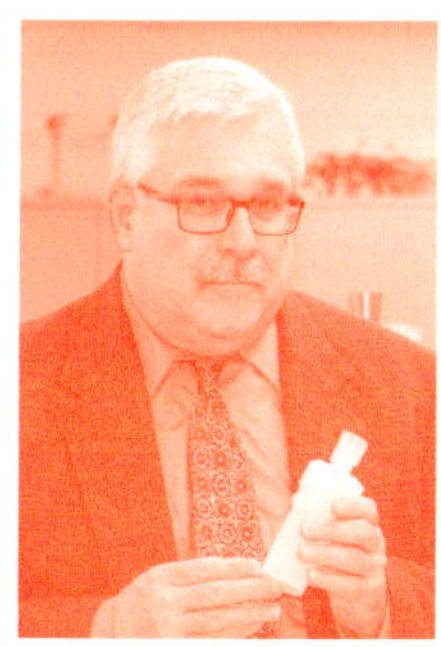
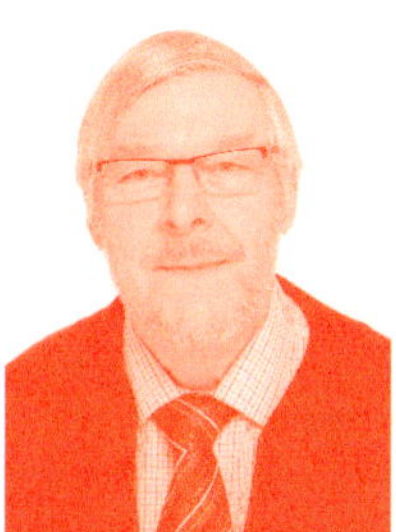
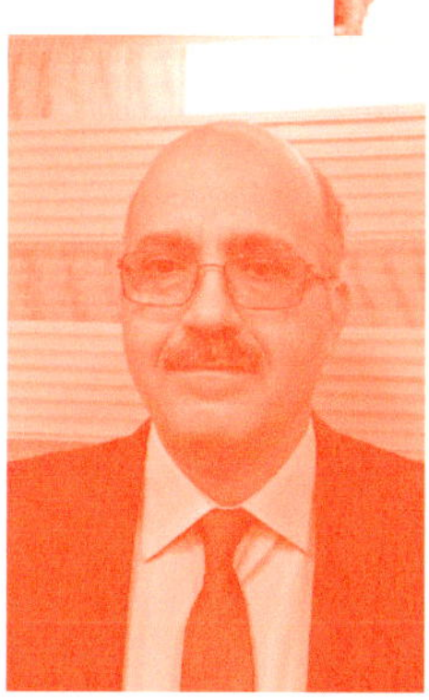
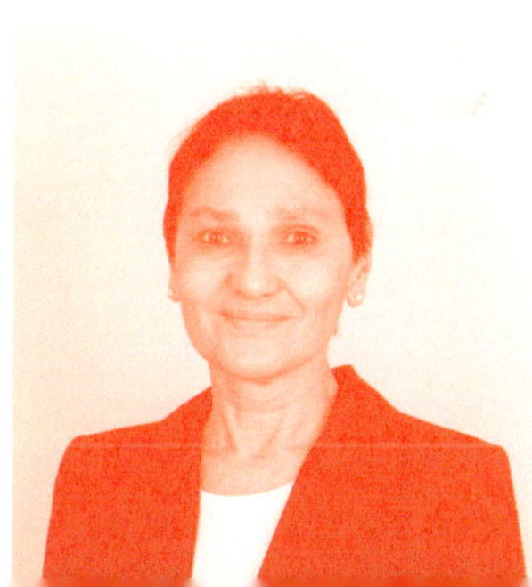
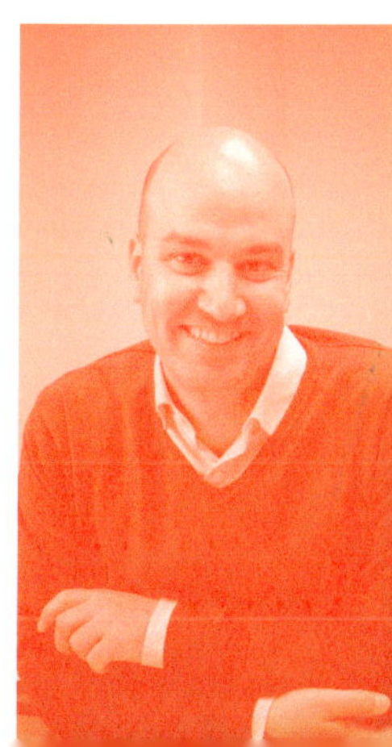

Neurodegenerative Diseases - Molecular Mechanisms and Current Therapeutic Approaches
http://dx.doi.org/10.5772/intechopen.83153
Edited by Nagehan Ersoy Tunalı

Contributors
Irina Kerkis, Eduardo Frare, Joyce Macedo Da Silva, Cristiane Valverde Wenceslau, Nicole Caroline Mambelli-Lisboa, Anoop Chakrapani, Maria Uscinska, Nicolo' Gagliano, Frank Ho-Yin Lai, Simote Foliaki, Cathryn Haigh, Bradley Groveman, Demet Özbabalık Adapınar, Oguz Erdinc, Demet Ilhan, Robin Warner, Kamil Kuca, Eugenie Nepovimova, Karla Isabel Lira-De León, Alma Delia Bertadillo-Jilote, David Gustavo García-Gutiérrez, Marco Meraz-Ríos, Ruchi Jakhmola-Mani, Deepshikha Pande Katare, Rajani Singh, Nagehan Ersoy Tunalı

First published in London, United Kingdom, 2021 by IntechOpen
IntechOpen is the global imprint of INTECHOPEN LIMITED, registered in England and Wales, registration number: 11086078, 5 Princes Gate Court, London, SW7 2QJ, United Kingdom
Printed in Croatia

British Library Cataloguing-in-Publication Data
A catalogue record for this book is available from the British Library

Additional hard and PDF copies can be obtained from orders@intechopen.com

Neurodegenerative Diseases - Molecular Mechanisms and Current Therapeutic Approaches
Edited by Nagehan Ersoy Tunalı
p. cm.
Print ISBN 978-1-83880-149-6
Online ISBN 978-1-83880-150-2
eBook (PDF) ISBN 978-1-83880-360-5

For EU product safety concerns:
IN TECH d.o.o., Prolaz Marije Krucifikse Kozulić 3, 51000 Rijeka, Croatia, info@intechopen.com or visit our website at intechopen.com.

Meet the editor

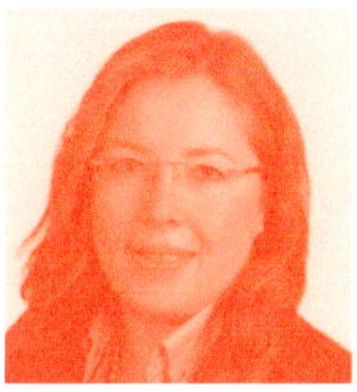

Nagehan Ersoy Tunalı received her Ph.D., M.Sc., and B.Sc. degrees in Molecular Biology and Genetics from the Boğaziçi University, İstanbul (TR). Her Ph.D. work involved "Molecular Analysis of Polyglutamine Diseases and Investigation of the Interaction Between Huntingtin and Nuclear Receptor Corepressor". She had the opportunity to gain experience in Huntington's Disease (HD) research at the University of Manchester (UK), CNR-Istituto di Medicina Sperimentale e Biotecnologie (IT) and the University of Wales College of Medicine (UK). She served as the Editor-in-Chief of the Journal of Cell and Molecular Biology between 2006 and 2016. Nagehan ERSOY TUNALI is currently conducting research on genetic modifiers of HD, localization and interactions of huntingtin, molecular mechanisms of excitotoxicity in HD, diagnostic biomarker discovery in AD, and nanotechnology-based therapeutic approaches in HD and AD.

Contents

Preface

Neurodegeneration is a broad term used to describe a range of processes that result in dysfunction and eventually death of the neurons. Neurodegenerative diseases represent a very large group of heterogeneous disorders affecting specific subtypes of neurons in the brain. Neurodegenerative diseases are listed among the leading causes of death and pose a serious public health challenge. Recently, the rising global burden of incurable neurodegenerative diseases has forced governments to allocate their financial and scientific resources to neurodegeneration research all around the world.

This book contributes both to the awareness of the anatomy and functions of our mysterious brain and its neurodegenerative states. In the first section of the book, our mini-brain, the cerebellum and its involvement in neurodegeneration are introduced first, since it has major roles in coordination, posture, balance, and important mental processes. In addition to that, the brain stress system and its contribution to neurodegeneration are discussed in a separate chapter. This section is finalized with a chapter involving biomarkers in emergency medicine and neurodegeneration, which will help clinicians and researchers search for certain emergency biomarkers in neurodegenerative conditions. The proceeding sections of the book include the presentation of three widely known and extensively studied neurodegenerative diseases; Alzheimer's Disease, Huntington's Disease, and Amyotrophic Lateral Sclerosis. The main molecular mechanisms, related biomarkers, and current modern therapy strategies are introduced. In addition to those, the characteristics of prion proteins in healthy cellular states and their involvement in prion diseases are discussed. In the last section of the book, molecular mechanisms of epilepsy are introduced, based on the fact that it is commonly associated with various neurodegenerative alterations in brain areas involved in electrographic seizures.

The book is intended to serve as a source to aid clinicians and researchers in the field, and also life science readers to increase their understanding and awareness of the clinical correlations, genetic aspects, neuropathological findings, and current therapeutic interventions in neurodegenerative diseases.

I would like to thank all the authors for their close cooperation and valuable work. I believe that this book will enlighten the curiosity for neurodegeneration and also encourage researchers to work on potentially effective molecular therapies for still mysterious neurodegenerative disorders.

Nagehan Ersoy Tunali, Ph.D.
Faculty of Engineering and Natural Sciences,
Department of Molecular Biology and Genetics,
İstanbul Medeniyet University,
İstanbul, Turkey

Section 1

Brain and Its Neurodegeneration

Chapter 1

Cerebellum: Its Anatomy, Functions and Diseases

Rajani Singh

Abstract

Cerebellum is the largest part of the hindbrain and weighs about 150 g. It is enshrined in posterior cranial fossa behind the pons and medulla oblongata and separated from these structures by cavity of fourth ventricle. It is connected to brainstem by three fibre tracts known as cerebellar peduncles. Cerebellum controls the same side of body. It precisely coordinates skilled voluntary movements by controlling strength, duration and force of contraction, so that they are smooth, balanced and accurate. It is also responsible for maintaining equilibrium, muscle tone and posture of the body. This is achieved through the use of somatic sensory information in modulating the motor output from the cerebrum and brainstem. Sherrington regarded cerebellum as the head ganglion of the proprioceptive system. Dysfunction of cerebellum along with degenerative diseases of cerebellum such as spinocerebellar ataxia, multiple sclerosis, malignant tumours, etc. may culminate into disequilibrium, hypotonia, difficulty in talking, sleeping, maintaining muscular coordination and dyssynergia which at times may be life threatening. Hence, knowledge of anatomy of cerebellum is imperative for neuroanatomists and neurosurgeons.

Keywords: cerebellum, pons, medulla, equilibrium, voluntary movements

1. Introduction

Cerebellum is a Latin word meaning little brain. It is the largest part of the hind brain and weighs about 150 g. It is enshrined in posterior cranial fossa beneath the

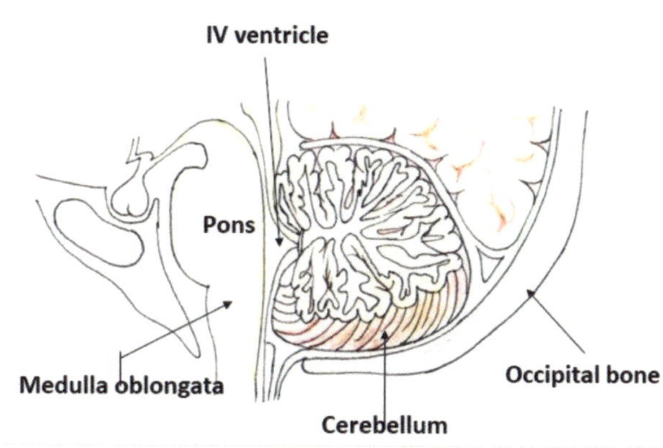

Figure 1.
The location and connections of cerebellum.

tentorium cerebelli behind the pons and medulla oblongata. Cerebellum is separated from the pons and medulla by the cavity of fourth ventricle (**Figure 1**).

Cerebellum is connected to brainstem by three large bundles of fibres called cerebellar peduncles. Superior peduncle connects cerebellum with mid brain, middle with pons and inferior with medulla oblongata [1].

2. Gross anatomy

Grossly cerebellum comprises of three parts: two surfaces, two notches and three well demarcated fissures (**Figure 2A** and **B**).

2.1 Parts

Cerebellum consists of two large bilateral lobes called cerebellar hemispheres. These two lobes are united to each other by a median worm like portion, vermis. Superior and inferior aspect of vermis are known as superior and inferior vermis, respectively. Superior vermis is continuous with the hemispheres but the inferior vermis is separated from hemispheres by deep furrow, the vallecular [2, 3].

2.2 Surfaces

Superior surface of the cerebellum is convex, and two cerebellar hemispheres are continuous with each other on this surface. Inferior surface presents deep furrow known as vallecular which separates two cerebellar hemispheres. The floor of the vallecular is occupied by inferior vermis.

2.3 Notches

There is a wide shallow gap known as anterior cerebellar notch on the anterior aspect of cerebellum. The anterior cerebellar notch lodges pons and medulla. Similarly, posteriorly there is posterior cerebellar notch which lodges falx cerebelli.

2.4 Fissures

Three fissures are related to cerebellum viz. horizontal, postero-lateral and primary fissures.

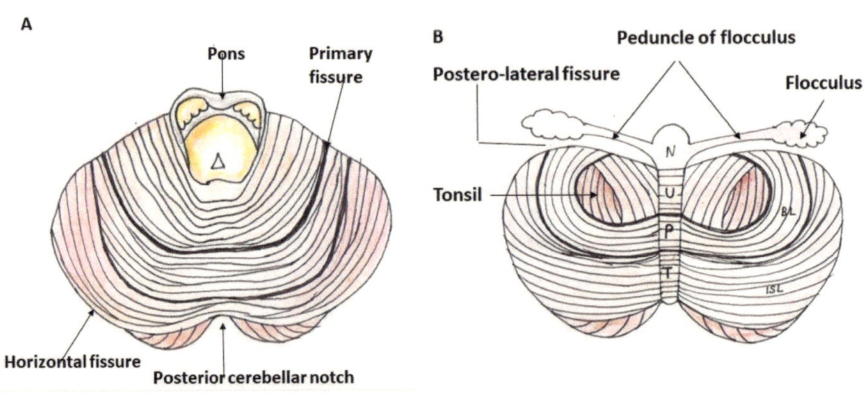

Figure 2.
(A) Schematic diagram showing superior surface of the cerebellum; (B) schematic diagram showing subdivisions of the cerebellum on the inferior surface. N = nodule, U = uvula, P = pyramid, T = tuber, BI = biventral lobule, ISL = inferior semilunar lobule.

Horizontal fissure is most prominent and courses along the lateral and posterior margins of the cerebellum. It separates the superior and inferior surfaces of the cerebellum.

Postero-lateral fissure is located on the inferior surface of the cerebellum and separates the flocculonodular lobe from the rest of the cerebellum also known as corpus cerebelli.

Primary fissure is situated on the superior surface and divides the corpus cerebelli into anterior and posterior (middle) lobes.

3. Subdivisions of cerebellum

3.1 Anatomical subdivisions

Cerebellum is divided by postero-lateral fissure into flocculonodular lobe and corpus cerebelli which is further divided by primary fissure into anterior and posterior lobes.

Flocculonodular lobe is located on the inferior surface in front of postero-lateral fissure and comprises of nodule of inferior vermis and a pair of floccule which are connected to the nodule by peduncles.

Anterior lobe is situated on the superior surface anterior to primary fissure. Vermal portion of anterior lobe consists of lingual, central lobule, and culmen.

Posterior lobe is located between the primary fissure on superior surface and postero-lateral fissure on inferior surface. This lobe includes both surfaces of cerebellum. Superior surface of posterior lobe consists of declive and folium while inferior surface consists of tuber, pyramid and uvula [4, 5].

Subdivisions of vermis and cerebellar hemispheres are described in **Table 1**.

Lobes	Subdivisions of vermis	Subdivisions of cerebellar hemispheres
Anterior lobe	Lingula	No lateral extension
	Central lobule	Ala
	Culmen	Quadrangular lobule
Posterior lobe	Declive	Lobulus simplex
	Folium	Superior semilunar lobule
	Tuber	Inferior semilunar lobule
	Pyramid	Biventral lobule
	Uvula	Tonsil
Flocculonodular lobe	Nodule	Flocculus

Table 1.
Subdivisions of vermis and cerebellar hemispheres.

4. Morphological subdivisions

Phylogenetically cerebellum is divided into three subdivisions: Archicerebellum, Paleocerebellum and Neocerebellum.

Archicerebellum (vestibular cerebellum): it is the oldest part of cerebellum and first to appear in aquatic vertebrates. Fishes and lower amphibians possess only this component of the cerebellum. Archicerebellum comprises of flocculonodular lobe and lingula and has mainly vestibular connections. It maintains equilibrium, tone and posture of trunk muscles.

Paleocerebellum (spinal cerebellum) appears next in terrestrial vertebrates with the appearance of limbs. It includes anterior lobe except lingula and pyramid and uvula. It is concerned with spinocerebellar connections and responsible for tone, posture and crude movements of the limbs.

Neocerebellum (cerebral cerebellum) is the most recent part of cerebellum to develop. It develops in primates and associated with the enlargement of telencephalone and cerebral cortex. It is very prominent in higher mammals. Neocerebellum includes posterior lobe except pyramid and uvula. It is mainly cortico-ponto-cerebellar connections and is concerned with smooth performance of skilled voluntary movements [4, 5].

5. Cytoarchitecture of cerebellum

Cerebellum consists of outer layer of grey matter, the cerebellar cortex and inner layer of white matter. Masses of grey matter, intracerebellar nuclei lie embedded in the white matter. Cerebellar cortex is folded to form narrow leaf like bands called folia. Each folium consists of central core of white matter surrounded by thin layer of grey matter. Central core of white matter is arranged in the form of the branching tree so called arbor vitae cerebelli.

5.1 Grey matter

Main features of grey matter are (a) cerebellar cortex and (b) intracebellar nuclei.

5.2 Structure of cerebellar

Cerebellar cortex composed of three distinct layers: (a) outer molecular layer, (b) intermediate Purkinje cell layer, and (c) inner granular layer cortex (**Figure 3**).

5.3 Molecular (plexiform) layer

This layer consists of unmyelinated nerve fibres derived from axons of granule, stellate and basket cells, dendrites of Purkinje and Golgi cells. It also contains

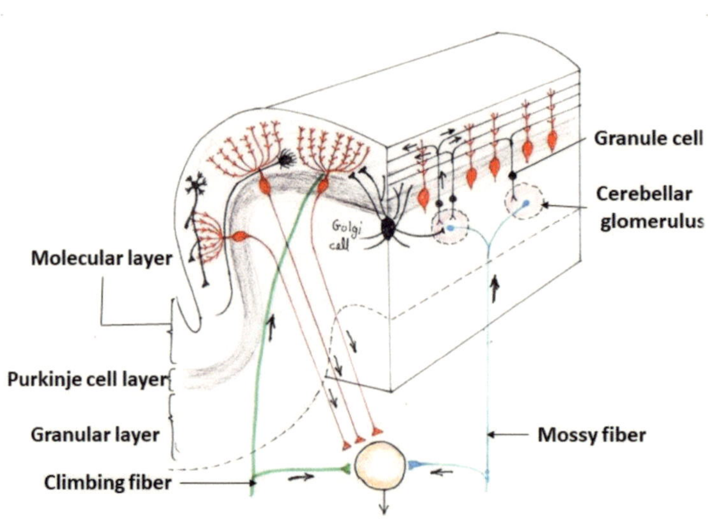

Figure 3.
Structure of cerebellar cortex along with intrinsic neurons and their processes.

stellate and basket cells. Stellate cells possess short process and are found scattered near the surface. The axons of these cell synapse with the dendrites of Purkinje cells. Basket cells contains little cytoplasm but have extensive processes. The axons of these cells follow transverse course parallel to the cortical surface and synapse with dendrites of Purkinje cells.

5.4 Purkinje cell layer

Purkinje cell layer consists of single layer of flask shaped Purkinje cells. Dendrites of these cells travel upwards into the molecular layer in which these cells undergo profuse branching. The dendrites of Purkinje cells synapse with collaterals of basket cells, axons of granule cells and climbing fibres. Axons of Purkinje cells travel through granular layer into white matter where they form synaptic connections with intracerebellar nuclei and exert inhibitory influence on these nuclei.

5.5 Granular layer

The inner granular layer composed of numerous granule cells and few Golgi cells. Each granule cell possesses 4–5 dendrites which synapse with mossy fibres. Axons of these cells courses into molecular layer where these bifurcates and branches pass parallel to the long axis of cerebellar folium. These fibres are known as parallel fibres and synapse with the dendrites of Purkinje cells.

Golgi cells are prominent but scanty, and their dendrites ramify in molecular layer.

Human cerebellum contains about 30–50 billion granule cells, 30 million Purkinje cells and 100 million stellate and basket cells. Purkinje cells, granule cells, stellate cells, basket cells and Golgi cells constitute intrinsic neurons of cerebellar cortex. All intrinsic neurons except granule cells are inhibitory and such collection of inhibitory neurons is not found anywhere in the central nervous system except cerebellum [1, 2].

6. Intracerebellar nuclei

Intracerebellar nuclei (**Figure 4**) also known as central nuclei are collection of grey matter embedded in white matter.

As these are situated close to roof of IV ventricle on each side of midline hence also referred as roof nuclei. From lateral to medial side, these are (1) Dentate nucleus, (2) Emboliform nucleus, (3) Globose nucleus, and (4) Fastigial nucleus.

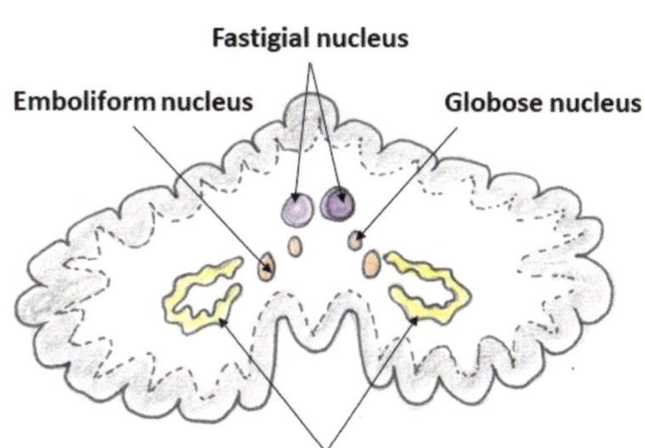

Figure 4.
Intracerebellar nuclei.

6.1 Dentate nucleus

It is the most prominent cerebellar nucleus and largest in primates including human beings. It belongs to neocerebellum and receives afferent from it. Its shape is like crumpled purse with hilum directed ventro-medially and its interior is filled with white matter consisting of efferent fibres forming most of the superior cerebellar peduncle.

6.2 Emboliform nucleus

It is oval shaped and located medial to dentate nucleus. It belongs to paleocerebellum, and this nucleus receives fibres from paleocerebellum and gives fibres to red nucleus via superior cerebellar peduncle.

6.3 Globose nucleus

It is rounded in shape and situated between emboliform and fastigial nuclei. It has similar connections as emboliform nucleus. Emboliform and globose nuclei together are known as nucleus interpositus.

6.4 Fastigial nucleus

This nucleus is situated in the midline in the vermis and smaller than dentate nucleus but larger than nucleus interpositus. It belongs to archicerebellum receiving afferents from it conveying efferents to vestibular and reticular nuclei.

7. White matter

White matter of cerebellum composed of three types of fibres viz. intrinsic, afferent and efferent. Intrinsic fibres are limited to cerebellum and connect different regions of cerebellum either of same hemispheres or of the two cerebellar hemispheres. Afferents and efferents connect cerebellum to other parts of central nervous system.

8. Connections of cerebellum

8.1 Afferent fibres

Cerebellum acquires information from cerebral cortex, spinal cord, vestibular apparatus, red nucleus and tectum of midbrain through afferent fibres. Cerebellum accrues input from cerebral cortex through cortico-ponto-cerebellar, cerebro-olivo-cerebellar and cerebro-reticulo-cerebellar pathways. Cerebellum receives information from spinal cord through anterior spinocerebellar, posterior spinocerebellar and cuneocerebellar tracts and that from vestibular apparatus either directly or after relaying in the vestibular nuclei [4, 5].

Afferent fibres reach the cerebellum through middle and inferior cerebellar peduncle and are of two types: (a) climbing fibres and (b) mossy fibres.

Climbing fibres arises in the inferior olivary nucleus and each fibre after giving a collateral to the intracerebellar nuclei synapses with the Purkinje cell. Mossy fibres are the main afferent fibres of cerebellum, and each mossy divides into 30–40 terminal swellings known as rosette which synapses with dendrites of granule cells and axons of Golgi cells. The structure formed by the rosette along with its synapses with granule and Golgi cells is known as cerebellar glomerulus which is spherical in shape surrounded by a capsule of neuroglial cells.

One climbing fibre synapses with single Purkinje cell; however, one mossy fibre synapses with many granule cells, and each granule cell synapses with thousands of Purkinje cells. Thus, one climbing fibre influences one Purkinje cells while one mossy fibres multitude of Purkinje cells. Both climbing and mossy fibres have excitatory effect on Purkinje cells.

8.2 Efferent fibres

Cerebellum provides output to red nucleus, thalamus, vestibular nuclei and reticular formation through efferent fibres via Purkinje cells. Majority of axons of Purkinje cells synapse with neurons of intracerebellar nuclei which in turn project to other parts of nervous system but few Purkinje cells from flocculonodular lobe and vermis directly end in lateral vestibular nuclei.

Efferent fibres from dentate, emboliform and globose nuclei travel through superior cerebellar peduncle and those from fastigial nucleus through inferior cerebellar peduncle.

9. Intrinsic cerebellar circuitry

All the afferent fibres to the cerebellum viz. climbing and mossy fibres are excitatory to the cells of cerebral cortex, and their collaterals are also excitatory to the intracerebellar nuclei. The climbing fibres excite the Purkinje cells directly but mossy fibres excite the Purkinje cells through granule cells which in turn excite basket and stellate cells but basket and stellate cells inhibit the Purkinje cells. Mossy fibres in addition also excite Golgi cells which in turn inhibit granule cells.

Purkinje cells inhibit intracerebellar nuclei which in turn control muscular activity through motor areas of brainstem and cerebral cortex.

10. Cerebellar peduncles

The afferent and efferent fibres of the cerebellum together form three bundles, cerebellar peduncles on each side. These peduncles are superior, middle and inferior.

Superior cerebellum connects cerebellum to the midbrain, middle to the pons and inferior to the medulla oblongata.

Superior cerebellar peduncle (brachium conjunctivum) ascends upward from the anterior cerebellar notch to the tectum of the midbrain. These peduncles form the supero-lateral boundary of the fourth ventricle. It conveys mainly efferent fibres from the cerebellum arising in dentate nucleus.

Middle cerebellar peduncle (brachium pontis) is the largest of three peduncles and consists principally of afferent fibres to the cerebellum. It bridges the basilar part of the pons and cerebellar hemispheres.

Inferior cerebellar peduncle (restiform body) connects dorso-lateral part of medulla oblongata and cerebellar hemispheres and composed of afferent fibres to the cerebellum from spinal cord, olivary nucleus, reticular formation of the medulla and vestibular nuclei.

11. Fibres transmitted by cerebellar peduncles

11.1 Superior cerebellar peduncle

This peduncle conveys both afferent and efferent fibres.

11.1.1 Afferent fibres

1. Anterior spino-cerebellar tract arise from the cells of laminae V-VII of the spinal cord. This tract convey proprioceptive and exteroceptive impulses from lower limb and lower part of the body and maintenance of posture and movement of lower limb.

2. Tecto-cerebellar tract originate from the superior and inferior colliculi of the midbrain tectum and are projected to the vermal and paravermal regions of declive, folium, tuber and pyramid and carry information from visual and auditory system.

3. Trigemino-cerebellar fibres arise from superior sensory and spinal nucleus of the trigeminal nerve and are projected to the culmen and declive.

4. Ceruleo-cerebellar is nor-adrenergic fibres arising from locus ceruleus and inhibiting Purkinje cells.

5. Hypothalamo-cerebellar fibres are cholinergic fibres originating from hypothalamus.

11.1.2 Efferent fibres

1. Dentato-thalamic fibres arise from dentate nucleus and projected to area 4 and 6 of the motor cortex regulating motor functions.

2. Cerebello-rubral fibres erupt from nucleus interpositus and end in contralateral red nucleus.

3. Cerebello-olivary fibres bud from dentate nucleus and terminate in inferior olivary nucleus.

4. Cerebello-reticular fibres originate from fastigial nucleus and end in reticular nuclei.

11.2 Middle cerebellar peduncle

11.2.1 Afferent fibres

1. Ponto-cerebellar fibres originate from pontine nuclei of basilar part of the pons and projected partly to contralateral neocerebellum and partly to contralateral paleocerebellum. Pontine nuclei receive fibres from cerebral cortex forming cerebro-ponto-cerebellar tract.

2. Reticulo-cerebellar tract arise from reticular formation of brainstem and are projected to the vermal region of the cerebellum.

3. Some serotonergic fibres from raphe nuclei of the pons reach the cerebellum through this peduncle.

11.2.2 Efferent fibres

No efferent fibres pass through this peduncle.

11.3 Inferior cerebellar peduncle

11.3.1 Afferent fibres

1. Posterior spino-cerebellar tract arises from thoracic nucleus (Clarke's column) of the spinal cord conveying proprioceptive and exteroceptive impulses from lower limb to paleocerebellum.

2. Cuneo-cerebellar tract (posterior external arcuate fibres) arise from ipsilateral accessory cuneate nucleus of medulla transmitting proprioceptive and exteroceptive impulses from upper limb and upper trunk and project on culmen and pyramid of vermis.

3. Anterior external arcuate fibres originate from arcuate nucleus of both sides and project into the neocerebellum.

4. Vestibulo-cerebellar tract primarily arise from vestibular nerve and secondary from medial and inferior vestibular nuclei forming juxta-restiform body and projecting to ipsilateral flocculonodular lobe, uvula and lingual. Few fibres end in fastigial nuclei.

5. Olivo-cerebellar tract sprout from contralateral inferior olivary nucleus and project into the neocerebellum but few fibres terminate into deep nuclei.

6. Parolivo-cerebellar tract arise from medial and dorsal accessory olivary nuclei and project on to the contralateral neocerebellum.

7. Reticulo-cerebellar tract buds from lateral and paramedian reticular nuclei of the medulla oblongata and project on to the neocerebellum.

11.3.2 Efferent fibres

1. Cerebello-vestibular fibres sprout from ipsilateral flocculonodular and fastigial nuclei of both sides. These fibres travel through juxta-restiform body and projected to vestibular nuclei

2. Cerebello-reticular fibres arise from fastigial nuclei of both sides and reaches the pontine and reticular formation. Fibres arising from contralateral fastigial nuclei form hook bundle of russel.

3. Cerebello-olivary fibre's origin is unknown and connect cerebellum with the inferior olivary nucleus.

12. Functions of cerebellum

1. Cerebellum maintains equilibrium, muscle tone, posture and coordinates skilled voluntary movements by regulating the grade of muscle tension between agonist and antagonist muscles.

2. Sherrington named cerebellum as the head ganglion of the proprioceptive system as various sensory inputs from the vestibular, visual and auditory systems, stretch receptors of muscle spindle and Golgi tendon organ, tactile and pressure receptors of head and body are relayed in the cerebellum. The sensory impulses are processed in the intrinsic cerebellar circuitry and integrated into the motor system by cerebral motor cortex, red nucleus, vestibular nuclei and reticular formation.

3. If the movement is to be carried out, cerebral cortex sends information to anterior horn cells of spinal cord to initiate movement, and it also sends impulses to cerebellum about the movement to be executed. Cerebellum also receives proprioceptive information from the muscles and joints about the actual movement occurring. The cerebellum compares both these information about movement and if any difference is noted in information concerning intended and actual movement, the cerebellum sends the information to cerebral cortex and anterior horn cells of the spinal cord to correct the discrepancy so that movement carried out is accurate in time, rate, range, force and direction.

13. Arterial supply of the cerebellum

The cerebellum is irrigated by three pairs of cerebellar arteries.

a. Superior cerebellar artery, branch of basilar artery irrigates superior surface of the cerebellum.

b. Anterior inferior cerebellar artery, branch of basilar artery supplies anterior part of inferior surface of cerebellum.

c. Posterior inferior cerebellar artery, branch of vertebral artery irrigates posterior part of inferior surface of cerebellum.

14. Applied anatomy

Cerebellar lesions may occur due to trauma, vascular occlusion, tumour or other pathologies producing cerebellar syndrome. Cerebellar syndrome is grouped in three types viz. Archicerebellar, paleocerebellar and neocerebellar syndromes.

14.1 Archicerebellar syndrome

In this syndrome, predominantly flocculonodular is affected by tumour, medulloblastoma. The patient is unable to maintain equilibrium while standing and falls on closing the eyes. This is called positive Romberg's sign. In addition to this, the patient walks on a wide base with legs well apart and sways from side to side.

14.2 Paleocerebellum syndrome

Lesion of this part of cerebellum produces hypotonia (decreased muscle tone) of limb muscles manifesting as:

a. Instability of joints resulting in flail joints.

b. Abnormal tendon reflex, for example, oscillating movements of leg are produced when patellar tendon is tapped (Pendular knee jerk).

c. Unable to maintain equilibrium while walking exhibiting ataxic gait.

14.3 Neocerebellum syndrome

Lesion in this part of cerebellum leads to incoordination known as asynergia and tremor which manifests in form of:

a. Ataxia due to incoordination of muscles of trunk, pectoral and pelvic girdles. The patient tends to fall on the side of lesion and to prevent fall patient stands or walk on a broad base.

b. Dysmetria culminates into past pointing where the patient is not able to measure the distance for performing intended task. This is tested by finger-nose test in which the patient is supposed to touch the tip of nose by finger but in this disorder the patient either over or under shoots the tip of nose.

c. Intention tremors appear during purposeful movements and disappear during rest. These tremors are coarse, arrhythmic and occur at the end of the movement.

d. Dysdiadochokinesis/adiadochokinesis is the inability to perform alternate movements with rapidity such as supination and pronation.

e. Rebound phenomenon occurs when the action of agonist muscle is not checked by corresponding antagonist muscle. If the patient is asked to push the palm of physician and when physician removes his hand, the hand of the patient moves back (rebounds) and hits the physician as the patient is unable to stop the pushing act immediately.

f. Dysarthria/scanning speech occurs due to incoordination of muscles responsible for speech. The speech is slurred, prolonged, explosive and with pauses at wrong places.

g. Nystagmus results in oscillation of eye ball due to incoordination of extraocular muscles.

In addition to above mentioned diseases, cerebellum is affected by certain neurodegenerative diseases which are elaborated below:

Cerebellar degenerative diseases:

a. **Spinocerebellar ataxia**

This condition involves mutation in genes causing degenerative changes in neurons of cerebellum including brainstem and spinal cord. If a parent is affected by this disease, there is 50% chance of inheriting the disease [6]. It is hereditary progressive degenerative disease often fatal. The disease is associated with progressive incoordination of gait, hand, speech and eye. No treatment is available only symptomatic relief can be provided to affected individuals.

b. **Multiple sclerosis**

In this condition, both genetic and environmental factors influence the outcome of diseases [7]. The myelin sheath enveloping the neurons is damaged resulting in delayed and interrupted impulses from and to the cerebellum [8]. It is incurable condition.

c. **Paraneoplastic disorders**

In this disorder, the person's autoimmune system especially T-cells become active in response to malignant tumours resulting in degeneration of neurons of cerebellum causing impaired ability to talk, walk, sleep, maintain balance and coordinate muscle activity [9]. This disorder is more common in middle aged individuals with lung, ovarian and breast cancer [10].

d. **Chronic alcohol abuse**

This condition is more prevalent in men than women. Chronic alcohol intake reduces vitamin B1 absorption and utilisation leading to degeneration of cerebellar neurons [11]. It is most common cause of nutritional spinocerebellar ataxia.

e. **Parkinson's disease**

Lesions of basal ganglion and cerebellum produce abnormal movements or changes in tone. Tremors occur both with the lesions of basal ganglion and cerebellum. However, tremors in cerebellar lesions occur only during movement, hence also known as intention tremors, while in basal ganglion diseases, like Parkinson's disease, tremors are observed during resting state. In addition to this, other signs of Parkinson's disease like mask face, clasp knife rigidity, lead pipe rigidity and hypokinesia/akinesia are not observed in cerebellar neurodegenerative diseases.

f. **Alzheimer's disease**

This chronic neurodegenerative disease is characterised by gradual onset of dementia. Alzheimer's disease is the cause of dementia in 60–70% cases. Most common early symptom is difficulty in remembering recent events [12]. Later on other symptoms like problems with language, disorientation and mood swings appear slowly. Though the causes of this disease can be various, the risk attributed to genetics is estimated to be around 70% [13]. In this disease, there is degeneration and loss of neurons and synapses in various parts of brain resulting in atrophy (reduction in size) of related regions. Amyloid plaques and neurofibrillary tangles are found deposited in the neurons of the brain [14].

g. **Huntington's disease**

Huntington's disease is also known as Huntington's chorea. It is an inherited disorder caused by mutation in the huntingtin gene which codes for huntingtin protein. Mutant huntingtin gene produces mutant and defective protein which is toxic to neurons of brain causing degenerative changes in brain. This causes problem with mood and mental abilities associated with lack of coordination and unsteady gait. Gradually coordinated movements become difficult and person is unable to talk [15]. There is as no treatment for the disease except for the supportive treatment.

15. Conclusion

Normally, cerebellum maintains equilibrium, muscle tone, posture and coordinates skilled voluntary movements which are very essential to carry out day to day activities. However, lesions of cerebellum may disrupt these actions which may cause various types of inconveniences and discomforts to the patients.

Dysfunction of cerebellum may culminate into disequilibrium, hypotonia and dyssynergia, which at times may be life threatening. In addition to the degenerative diseases of cerebellum described above, it causes difficulty in talking eating, sleeping coordination of muscular activity and other neurological complications. Hence, knowledge of the anatomy of the cerebellum is imperative for neuroanatomists and neurosurgeons.

DOI: http://dx.doi.org/10.5772/intechopen.93064

Author details

Rajani Singh
Department of Anatomy, UP University of Medical Sciences Saifai Etawah, UP, India

*Address all correspondence to: nani_sahayal@rediffmail.com

References

[1] Standring S. Gray's Anatomy Chapter-the Cerebellum. 39th ed. Edinberg: Churchill Livinstone; 2005. pp. 353-368

[2] Datta AK. Essentials of Human Anatomy-Neuroanatomy, Chapter- the Cerebellum. 4th ed. India (Kolkata): Current Books International; 2013. pp. 166-181

[3] Singh V. Textbook of Clinical Neurotomy Chapter-the Cerebellum. 2nd ed. India (New Delhi): Elsevier; 2011. pp. 111-119

[4] Chaurasia BD. Human Anatomy (Head Neck and Brain) Chapter-Cerebellum. 4th ed. India (New Delhi): CBS Publishers and distributors; 2009. pp. 389-394

[5] Kulkarni NV. Clinical Anatomy Chapter-Cerebellum. 2nd ed. India (New Delhi): Jaypee Brothers. 2012. pp. 532-535

[6] Ataxias and Cerebellar or Spinocerebellar Degeneration Information Page. National Institute of Neurological Disorders and Stroke. Available from: https://www.ninds.nih.gov/Disorders/All-Disorders/Ataxias-and-Cerebellar-or-Spinocerebellar-Degeneration-Information-Page

[7] Lublin FD, Reingold SC, Cohen JA, et al. Defining the clinical course of multiple sclerosis: The 2013 revisions. Neurology. 2013;**83**(3):278-286

[8] Biologydictionary.net Editors. "Myelin Sheath." Biology Dictionary, Biologydictionary.net. 2017. Available from: https://biologydictionary.net/myelin-sheath/

[9] Paraneoplastic syndromes of the nervous system - Symptoms and causes. Mayo Clinic. 2020. [Accessed: 5th May 2020]

[10] NINDS Paraneoplastic Syndromes Information Page. National Institute of Neurological Disorders and Stroke Website. 2009. Available from: https://www.ninds.nih.gov/Disorders/All-Disorders/Paraneoplastic-Syndromes-Information-Page [Accessed: 5th May 2020]

[11] Shanmugarajah PD, Hoggard N, Currie S, Aeschlimann DP, Aeschlimann PC, Gleeson DC, et al. Alcohol-related cerebellar degeneration: Not all down to toxicity? Cerebellum & Ataxias. 2016;**3**(1):17

[12] Burns A, Iliffe S. Alzheimer's disease. BMJ. 2009;**338**:b158. DOI: 10.1136/bmj.b158

[13] Ballard C, Gauthier S, Corbett A, Brayne C, Aarsland D, Jones E. Alzheimer's disease. Lancet. 2011;**377**(9770):1019-1031

[14] Wenk GL. Neuropathologic changes in Alzheimer's disease. The Journal of Clinical Psychiatry. 2003;**64**(Suppl 9):7-10

[15] Dayalu P, Albin RL. Huntington disease: Pathogenesis and treatment. Neurologic Clinics. 2015;**33**(1):101-114. DOI: 10.1016/j.ncl.2014.09.003

Chapter 2

The Brain Stress System in the Neurobiology of the "Dark Side" of Addiction and Its Relation to Neurodegeneration

Maria Uscinska, Nicolo' Gagliano and Frank Ho-Yin Lai

Abstract

Addiction is a chronically relapsing disorder characterized by a compulsion to seek and take a substance of abuse, the development of dependence, and a negative emotional state when intake is stopped. Compelling evidence argues that dysregulation of the brain stress system is a key constituent of the addiction process. Through mechanisms of negative reinforcement, the stress system is posited to induce negative emotional state referred to as the 'dark side of addiction' as it becomes the powerful motivation for drug-seeking associated with compulsive use. Therein, the neuropharmacological actions of corticotropin-releasing factor (CRF) is posited to play a key role in the anxiety/stress-like effects of acute withdrawal, anxiety/stress-like effects of abstinence, and relapse to drug taking. In this view, the present chapter sheds a critical light on latest research developments implicating this largely neglected component of substance abuse to give insight into the neuropathology of the 'dark side' of addiction. Moreover, the chapter provides insight into individual vulnerability to addiction and proposes a novel treatment candidate for the disorder.

Keywords: addiction, stress, neurobiology, corticotropin-releasing factor, hypothalamic-pituitary-adrenal (HPA) axis

1. Conceptual framework

DSM-5 defines addiction as an evolving and chronically relapsing disorder, characterized by a compulsion to take drugs, the development of dependence and a motivational withdrawal syndrome with a negative emotional state when access to the drug is prevented [1, 2]. The profound malaise and anxiety during withdrawal, protracted abstinence syndrome marked by a low-level anxiety/dysphoria, and a high vulnerability to relapse upon exposure to an acute stressor is aptly termed 'the dark side' of addiction. It is the common element of the disorder, although all addictions to different drugs are characterized by distinct patterns with emphasis on different stages of the addiction cycle.

The disorder typically progresses in a cyclical manner through three stages, namely preoccupation/anticipation, binge/intoxication, and withdrawal/negative affect (see **Figure 1**). The early stages of the cycle are characterized by impulsivity,

IntechOpen

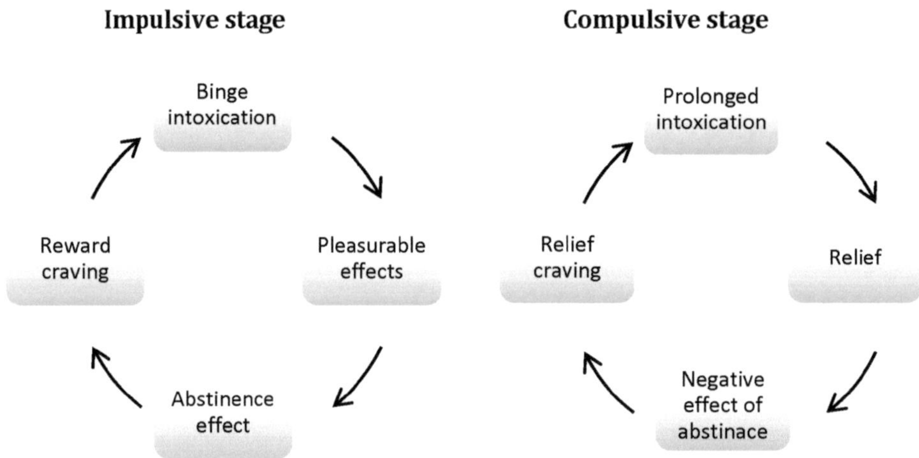

Figure 1.
The progression of alcohol dependence over time marked by a shift in underlying motivational mechanisms. From initial, positively reinforcing, pleasurable drug effects, the addictive process progresses over time to being driven by negatively reinforcing relief from a negative emotional state.

whereas terminal stages are dominated by compulsivity. The former refers to rapid reactions to internal and external factors with no concern about negative outcomes whilst the latter to perseveration in actions despite adverse consequences or in the face of incorrect responses in choice situations. As the cycle of drug taking and withdrawal continues, the different components of the addiction cycle become more intense, and progressively evolve into a more severe pathology [1]. This process is accompanied by changes in the motivational behavioral mechanism that maintains addiction. Inasmuch as removal of negative emotional state associated with drug withdrawal becomes the mechanism driving the dependence-induced drug intake, there is a shift from positive to negative reinforcement maintaining the motivated behavior [3].

2. The dark side of addiction

In relation to the dark side of addiction, a wealth of data supports that symptoms of acute withdrawal from chronic drugs of abuse tend to be affective in nature, persist beyond the acute phase to protracted abstinence, and precede relapse to drug-seeking [4, 5]. Tension, fatigue and anxiety related to alcohol withdrawal have been shown to last from 5 to 9 months post-withdrawal [6, 7]. Furthermore, negative affective symptoms appear to be the leading precipitant of relapse [8, 9]. By way of example, the association between relapse and a subclinical negative affective state was shown to be particularly strong in patients with alcohol dependence, who underwent a 12-week clinical trial [10]. Animal data further shows that a history of dependence lowers the "dependence threshold" and makes the subsequent addiction more severe, relative to subjects receiving alcohol for the first time [11–14]. Moreover, the former category evidenced a prolonged elevation in ethanol self-administration after acute withdrawal and detoxification [15–18], and this was accompanied by increased overt responsivity to stressors and increased responsivity to antagonists of the brain CRF systems [19–21]. Finally, evidence exists to support that a history of prior dependence increases sensitivity to stress-induced reinstatement upon exposure to variety of stressors such as footshock, social stress, or pharmacological stress (e.g., yohimbine) [22]. Notably, the neural mechanism of stress-induced reinstatement overlaps with that of acute motivational withdrawal [23]. In what follows, next sections of the chapter provide a conceptual framework linking addiction to stress systems.

3. Brain stress systems and addiction

In neural terms, the "dark side" of addiction is posited to be mediated by activation of brain stress system that interacts with hormonal stress systems. Emerging evidence have highlighted that dysregulation of brain arousal/stress systems plays a key role in pathophysiology of drug addiction [2]. More relevant to this chapter, the negative emotional state associated with the dark side of addiction has been linked to a cycle of increasing dysregulation of brain reward/anti-reward mechanisms. Therein, corticotropin releasing factor (CRF) appears to be the prominent component of the negative reinforcement processes that drive the compulsivity of addiction [2].

CRF is a 41-amino acid polypeptide that mobilizes the body's hormonal, autonomic, and behavioral responses to stressors (for a review of the biology of CRF systems see [24, 25]). It has a wide distribution across the brain with particularly high concentrations of cell bodies in the paraventricular nucleus of the hypothalamus, the basal forebrain, and the brainstem [26]. Therein, majority of stress-like effects are mediated by the brain and pituitary CRF_1 receptors [25]. The urocortin/CRF_2 systems have been less explored, with some data pointing to neuroadaptation associated with chronic drug use, also in opposition to the effects of the CRF_1 receptor.

Initial drug use at the binge/intoxication stage of addiction cycle activates the hypothalamic pituitary-adrenal (HPA) axis, which initiates acquisition of drug-seeking behavior through activity in the brain motivational circuits [27–30]. HPA axis activity is characterized by a cascade of physiological changes within the paraventricular nucleus of the hypothalamus, the anterior lobe of the pituitary gland, and the adrenal gland (for review, see Ref. [31]).

The CRF is synthesized by neurosecretory neurons in the medial parvocellular subdivision of the paraventricular nucleus and released into the portal blood vessels of the anterior pituitary gland. Therein it binds to the CRF_1 receptor on pituitary corticotropes triggering the release of adreno-corticotropin hormone (ACTH) into the systemic circulation, which induces glucocorticoid synthesis and secretion from the adrenal cortex.

Once drug-seeking behavior is initiated, the transition from acute to chronic administration of drugs of abuse is mediated by progressive changes in the HPA axis that can lead to subsequent activation of extrahypothalamic brain stress systems characterizing the withdrawal/negative affect stage [32–34]. The HPA axis is regulated via negative feedback from circulating glucocorticoids that act on glucocorticoid receptors in the paraventricular nucleus and the hippocampus. Although high levels of glucocorticoids can feedback to shut off the HPA axis, they can also sensibilize CRF systems in the central nucleus of the amygdala and basolateral amygdala involved in behavioral responses to stressors [35–39]. This observation lends support to the thesis that CRF has a key role in the dark side of the addiction process.

4. Allostatic model of addiction

As the cycle of drug taking and withdrawal continues, the different components of the addiction cycle become more intense, changes also the motivational behavioral mechanism that maintains addiction. The shift from positive to negative reinforcement behind motivation in compulsive drug use might be explained by allostatic model of the brain motivational systems. It defines addiction as a failure of counteradaptive processes of optimal homeostatic reward functioning to return to their normal range [2, 40]. Therein, the posited mechanism of pathology is mediated by within-system neuroadaptations (changes in reward pathways) and between-system neuroadaptations (brain stress systems) [1, 41].

The body's response to stress related to addiction is controlled by CRF in the paraventricular nucleus of the hypothalamus. It maintains homeostasis by orchestrating rapid and sustained responses to anticipated challenges to normal operating level of the regulatory system. Upon exposure to an environmental challenge, a feed-forward mechanism continuously re-evaluates the environmental demand for adaption, and accordingly readjusts all parameters toward new set points to mobilize resources quickly. However, it might become the engine for pathology if insufficient resources are available to shut off the response. This leads to an allostatic state, defined as a stability with an altered set point [42]. In this view, CRF becomes the key contributor to allostasis and it is hypothesized to mediate the compulsivity and relapse to drug-seeking and drug-taking in addiction [43].

More relevant to this treatise, repeated administration of drugs of abuse leads to an alteration in psychological homeostatic processes, characterized by overactivation of normal arousal or emotional systems in the body [44]. Given that addiction shares some common characteristic with chronic physiological disorders, it allows to speculate that it represents a chronic deviation of the regulatory system from its normal operating level, rather than mere homeostatic dysregulation of emotional function.

Just like any chronic physiological disorder, addiction is subject to significant environmental stressors, deteriorates with time, and is marked by a residual neural trace for rapid re-addiction even after years of abstinence. In response to excessive drug use the brain attempts to maintain homeostatic stability through molecular, cellular, and neurocircuitry changes that occur at the cost of allostatic state. Allostasis represents a chronic deviation from optimal brain emotional regulation marked by decreased function of reward circuits, strengthened stimulus–response associations, loss of executive control and recruitment of the brain stress systems. These neurobiological changes underpin the chronic elevation of reward threshold associated with negative emotional state, thereby contributing to the compulsive drug use [45]. In this view, the cycle of increasing dysregulation of brain reward/anti-reward mechanisms constitutes the posited mechanism of the negative emotions in addiction and compulsive drug use.

5. CRF in the dark side of addiction

All drugs of abuse activate the HPA axis during acquisition of drug-taking and acute withdrawal from the drug by releasing CRF in the paraventricular nucleus of the hypothalamus. Activation of the axis during acute administration facilitates activity in the brain motivational circuits of drug reward, thereby promoting acquisition of drug-seeking behavior [27–30]. Repeated administration dysregulates these acute changes beyond HPA axis to affect the brain extrahypothalamic stress system [46–49]. Therein the repeated exposure to high levels of glucorticoids may have profound effects on the extrahypothalamic brain stress systems, contributing to the persistence and relapse to cycles of addiction to drugs of abuse [32]. Repeated addiction cycles not only blunt the HPA axis response but also sensitize the response of the extrahypothalamic CRF stress system in the amygdala [34]. Whilst initially the presence of glucocorticoids enhances response to novelty and reward, sensitization of CRF systems in the extended amygdala may contribute to a stress component of the shift from homeostasis to pathophysiology of drug addiction. The stress component is posited to constitute an opponent anti-reward process response to excessive activation of reward systems [2].

Compelling evidence exist to support the thesis that the neuroanatomical substrates for many of the motivational effects associated with the dark side of addiction constitute a common neural circuitry within the basal forebrain, termed the "extended amygdala" [50]. It represents a macrostructure comprising the bed nucleus of the stria terminalis, central medial amygdala, and a transition zone in the posterior part of the medial nucleus accumbens (i.e., posterior shell) [51, 52]. Importantly, the extended amygdala includes dopamine and opioid peptides associated with the positive reinforcing effects of drugs of abuse, and major components of the extrahypothalamic CRF systems associated with negative reinforcement mechanisms [33]. It receives afferent connections from limbic cortices, the hippocampus, basolateral amygdala, midbrain, and lateral hypothalamus and efferent connections to the posterior medial ventral pallidum, ventral tegmental area, various brainstem projections, and to the lateral hypothalamus [52]. The arousal/stress brain systems in the extended amygdala may play a key role in the negative emotional states that maintains addiction to drugs of abuse and may overlap with the negative emotional constituent of other psychopathologies.

6. Brain stress and neurodegeneration

Stress might exert either ameliorating or detrimental effects on physiological processes. In the short term it might be beneficial to an organism however in the long-term it plays a major role in various pathophysiology related to neurodegenerative diseases and mood disorders. Upon exposure to stress the body enters the 'fight or flight' stage, after which it builds resistance to the stress in the adaptation stage, and finally due to 'wear and tear' it reaches exhaustion [53]. In the adaptation stage, cortisol typically exerts a negative feedback effect to shut down the stress response. Multiple brain regions related to cognition are actively involved in feedback regulation including the hippocampus, amygdala, the brain stem and prefrontal cortex [54]. Accordingly, stimulation by corticosteroids induced at the level of the amygdala, the prefrontal cortex and the locus coeruleus was found to interfere with HPA activity and memory [55]. A deficient cortisol feedback effect caused by glucocorticoid resistance increases the activity of the HPA-axis have been found to be associated with neurodegenerative diseases, obesity, heart disease, depression, and a variety of other health issues [56]. Therein the vasopressin neurons of the central nervous system inhibit the regulatory influence of CRH neurons in the PVN resulting in a disproportionally high activity of the HPA system.

Given the inhibitory control of the hippocampus over the HPA-axis, damage to this structure is posited to be causally involved in disinhibition of the HPA axis activity thereby accounting for the age-related accumulation of hippocampal damage in Alzheimer's disease (AD) and depression. This thesis is furthered by evidence of increased cortisol plasma levels in early stage of AD associated with cognitive decline [57], and a correlation of salivary cortisol levels with the severity of the disease [58]. Accordingly, neuronal atrophy was evidenced in the hippocampus of stressed or corticosteroid-treated rodents and primates [59]. Elevated CRH and cortisol levels were also shown to contribute to the symptoms of depression in a large subpopulation of depressed subjects [56]. This is corroborated by the normalizing effect of antidepressants on the synthesis of CRH by stimulation and/or upregulation of corticosteroid receptor expression, and reversal the clinical symptoms [60]. In light of these evidence, the 'glucocorticoid cascade hypothesis' is posited to be the dominant pathogenetic mechanism in human neurodegenerative diseases marked by HPA-axis alterations including depression and AD [61].

Although CRH and cortisol seem to be etiologically involved in the development of depression, conclusive arguments cannot be drawn due to no evidence for any major damage in the human hippocampus in the disorder. Moreover, reduced hippocampal volume does not necessarily translate in cell death and might alternatively be explained by changes is water content or the structure in glial cells.

7. Summary and conclusions

Addiction to all drugs of abuse involves activation of the HPA axis. Pathophysiology of drug addiction involves dysregulation of the brain emotional system posited to be a key constituent of the negative emotional state produced by dependence that maintains drug-seeking through the mechanism of negative reinforcement. More specifically, the action of CRF in extra hypothalamic systems in the extended amygdala is considered a neural substrate of the pathophysiology of the disorder and plays a key role in maintaining the addiction cycle once it is initiated. It comprises the central nucleus of the amygdala, bed nucleus of the stria terminalis, and a transition area in the shell of the nucleus accumbens. Beyond providing insight into the neurobiology of the dark side of addiction, better characterization of the CRF systems in addiction hold promise for new targets for identifying vulnerability to addiction and novel treatments for the disorder.

Conflict of interest

The author has no relevant affiliations or financial involvement with any organization or entity with a financial interest in or financial conflict with the subject matter or materials discussed in the manuscript. This includes employment, consultancies, honoraria, stock ownership or options, expert testimony, grants or patents received or pending, or royalties. No writing assistance was utilized in the production of this manuscript.

Author details

Maria Uscinska[1*], Nicolo' Gagliano[2] and Frank Ho-Yin Lai[3]

1 Department of Neurosciences, University of Turin, Centre for Personality Disorders, Turin, Italy

2 Humanitas Research Hospital, Milan, Italy

3 Rehabilitation Sciences, Hong Kong Polytechnic University, Hong Kong

*Address all correspondence to: actapsy@gmail.com

References

[1] Koob GF, Le Moal M. Drug abuse: Hedonic homeostatic dysregulation. Science. 1997;**278**:52-58. DOI: 10.1126/science.278.5335.52

[2] Koob GF, Le Moal M. Addiction and the brain antireward system. Annual Review of Psychology. 2008;**59**:29-53. DOI: 10.1146/annurev.psych.59.103006.093548

[3] Koob GF. Allostatic view of motivation: Implications for psychopathology. In: Bevins RA, Bardo MT, editors. Motivational Factors in the Etiology of Drug Abuse. Nebraska Symposium on Motivation. Vol. 50. Lincoln, NE: University of Nebraska Press; 2004. pp. 1-18

[4] Hershon HI et al. Alcohol withdrawal symptoms and drinking behavior. Journal of Studies on Alcohol. 1977;**38**:953-971. DOI: 10.15288/jsa.197738.953

[5] Annis HM, Sklar SM, Moser AE. Gender in relation to relapse crisis situations, coping, and outcome among treated alcoholics. Addictive Behaviors. 1998;**23**:127-131. DOI: 10.1016/s0306-4603(97)00024-5

[6] Roelofs SM. Hyperventilation, anxiety, craving for alcohol: A subacute alcohol withdrawal syndrome. Alcohol. 1985;**2**:501-505. DOI: 10.1016/0741-8329(85)90123-5

[7] Alling C, Balldin J, Bokstrom K, Gottfries CG, Karlsson I, Langstrom G. Studies on duration of a late recovery period after chronic abuse of ethanol: A cross-sectional study of biochemical and psychiatric indicators. Acta Psychiatrica Scandinavica. 1982;**66**: 384-397. DOI: 10.1111/j.1600-0447.1982.tb06720.x

[8] Zywiak WH, Connors GJ, Maisto SA, Westerberg VS. Relapse research and the Reasons for Drinking Questionnaire: A factor analysis of Marlatt's relapse taxonomy. Addiction. 1996;**91**(Suppl):S121-S130. PMID: 8997786

[9] Lowman C, Allen J, Stout RL. Replication and extension of Marlatt's taxonomy of relapse precipitants: Overview of procedures and results. The Relapse Research Group. Addiction. 1996;**91**(Suppl):S51-S71. PMID: 8997781

[10] Mason BJ, Ritvo EC, Morgan RO, Salvato FR, Goldberg G, Welch B, et al. A double-blind, placebo-controlled pilot study to evaluate the efficacy and safety of oral nalmefene HCl for alcohol dependence. Alcoholism, Clinical and Experimental Research. 1994;**18**:1162-1167. DOI: 10.1111/j.1530-0277.1994.tb00098.x

[11] Branchey M, Rauscher G, Kissin B. Modifications in the response to alcohol following the establishment of physical dependence. Psychopharmacologia. 1971;**22**:314-322. DOI: 10.1007/bf00406870

[12] Baker TB, Cannon DS. Potentiation of ethanol withdrawal by prior dependence. Psychopharmacology. 1979;**60**:105-110. DOI: 10.1007/bf00432279

[13] Becker HC, Hale RL. Ethanol-induced locomotor stimulation in C57BL/6 mice following RO154513 administration. Psychopharmacology. 1989;**99**:333-336. DOI: 10.1007/bf00445553

[14] Becker HC. Positive relationship between the number of prior ethanol withdrawal episodes and the severity of subsequent withdrawal seizures. Psychopharmacology. 1994;**116**:26-32. DOI: 10.1007/bf02244867

[15] Roberts AJ, Heyser CJ, Cole M, Griffin P, Koob GF. Excessive ethanol

drinking following a history of dependence: Animal model of allostasis. Neuropsychopharmacology. 2000;**22**:581-594. DOI: 10.1016/S0893-133X(99)00167-0

[16] Rimondini R, Arlinde C, Sommer W, Heilig M. Long-lasting increase in voluntary ethanol consumption and transcriptional regulation in the rat brain after intermittent exposure to alcohol. The FASEB Journal. 2002;**16**:27-35. DOI: 10.1096/fj.01-0593com

[17] Rimondini R, Sommer WH, Dall'Olio R, Heilig M. Long-lasting tolerance to alcohol following a history of dependence. Addiction Biology. 2008;**13**:26-30. DOI: 10.1111/j.1369-1600.2007.00079.x

[18] Sommer WH, Rimondini R, Hansson AC, Hipskind PA, Gehlert DR, et al. Upregulation of voluntary alcohol intake, behavioral sensitivity to stress, and amygdala crhr1 expression following a history of dependence. Biological Psychiatry. 2008;**63**:139-145. DOI: 10.1016/j.biopsych.2007.01.010

[19] Valdez GR, Zorrilla EP, Roberts AJ, Koob GF. Antagonism of corticotropin-releasing factor attenuates the enhanced responsiveness to stress observed during protracted ethanol abstinence. Alcohol. 2003;**29**:55-60. DOI: 10.1016/s0741-8329(03)00020-x

[20] Valdez GR, Sabino V, Koob GF. Increased anxiety-like behavior and ethanol self-administration in dependent rats: Reversal via corticotropin-releasing factor-2 receptor activation. Alcoholism, Clinical and Experimental Research. 2004;**28**:865-872. DOI: 10.1097/01.alc.0000128222.29875.40

[21] Gehlert DR, Cippitelli A, Thorsell A, Le AD, Hipskind PA, et al. 3-(4-Chloro-2-morpholin-4-yl-thiazol-5-yl)-8-(1-ethylpropyl)2,6-dimethyl-imidazo[1,2-b] pyridazine: A novel brain-penetrant, orally available corticotropin-releasing factor receptor 1 antagonist with efficacy in animal models of alcoholism. The Journal of Neuroscience. 2007;**27**:2718-2726. DOI: 10.1523/JNEUROSCI.4985-06.2007

[22] Liu X, Weiss F. Additive effect of stress and drug cues on reinstatement of ethanol seeking: Exacerbation by history of dependence and role of concurrent activation of corticotropin-releasing factor and opioid mechanisms. The Journal of Neuroscience. 2002;**22**:7856-7861. PMCID: PMC6758095

[23] Shaham Y, Shalev U, Lu L, de Wit H, Stewar J. The reinstatement model of drug relapse: History, methodology and major findings. Psychopharmacology. 2003;**168**:3-20. DOI: 10.1007/s00213-002-1224-x

[24] Bale TL, Vale WW. CRF and CRF receptors: Role in stress responsivity and other behaviors. Annual Review of Pharmacology and Toxicology. 2004;**44**:525-557. DOI: 10.1146/annurev.pharmtox.44.101802.121410

[25] Heinrichs SC, Menzaghi F, Schulteis G, Koob GF, Stinus L. Suppression of corticotropin-releasing factor in the amygdala attenuates aversive consequences of morphine withdrawal. Behavioural Pharmacology. 1995;**6**:74-80. PMID: 11224314

[26] Swanson LW, Sawchenko PE, Rivier J, Vale W. The organization of ovine corticotropin-releasing factor immunoreactive cells and fibers in the rat brain: An immunohistochemical study. Neuroendocrinology. 1983;**36**:165-186. DOI: 10.1159/000123454

[27] Piazza PV, Deroche V, Deminiere JM, Maccari S, Le Moal M, Simon H. Corticosterone in the range of stress-induced levels possesses reinforcing properties: Implications

for sensation-seeking behaviors. Proceedings of the National Academy of Sciences of the United States of America. 1993;**90**:11738-11742. DOI: 10.1073/pnas.90.24.11738

[28] Piazza PV, Le Moal M. Glucocorticoids as a biological substrate of reward: Physiological and pathophysiological implications. Brain Research Reviews. 1997;**25**:359-372. DOI: 10.1016/s0165-0173(97)00025-8

[29] Goeders NE. A neuroendocrine role in cocaine reinforcement. Psychoneuroendocrinology. 1997;**22**:237-259. DOI: 10.1016/s0306-4530(97)00027-9

[30] Fahlke C, Hard E, Hansen S. Facilitation of ethanol consumption by intracerebroventricular infusions of corticosterone. Psychopharmacology. 1996;**127**:133-139. DOI: 10.1007/BF02805986

[31] Smith SM, Vale WW. The role of the hypothalamic-pituitary-adrenal axis in neuroendocrine responses to stress. Dialogues in Clinical Neuroscience. 2006;**8**:383-395. PMCID: PMC3181830

[32] Kreek MJ, Koob GF. Drug dependence: Stress and dysregulation of brain reward pathways. Drug and Alcohol Dependence. 1998;**51**:23-47. DOI: 10.1016/s0376-8716(98)00064-7

[33] Koob GF, Le Moal M. Plasticity of reward neurocircuitry and the 'dark side' of drug addiction. Nature Neuroscience. 2005;**8**:1442-1444. DOI: 10.1038/nn1105-1442

[34] Koob GF, Kreek MJ. Stress, dysregulation of drug reward pathways, and the transition to drug dependence. American Journal of Physics. 2007;**17**:24-49. DOI: 10.1176/appi.ajp.2007.05030503

[35] Imaki T, Nahan JL, Rivier C, Sawchenko PE, Vale W. Differential regulation of corticotropin-releasing factor mRNA in rat brain regions by glucocorticoids and stress. The Journal of Neuroscience. 1991;**11**:585-599. PMCID: PMC6575358

[36] Makino S, Gold PW, Schulkin J. Corticosterone effects on corticotropin-releasing hormone mRNA in the central nucleus of the amygdala and the parvocellular region of the paraventricular nucleus of the hypothalamus. Brain Research. 1994;**640**:105-112. DOI: 10.1016/0006-8993(94)91862-7

[37] Swanson LW, Simmons DM. Differential steroid hormone and neural influences on peptide mRNA levels in CRH cells of the paraventricular nucleus: A hybridization histochemical study in the rat. The Journal of Comparative Neurology. 1989;**285**:413-435. DOI: 10.1002/cne.902850402

[38] Schulkin J, McEwen BS, Gold PW. Allostasis, amygdala, and anticipatory angst. Neuroscience and Biobehavioral Reviews. 1994;**18**:385-396. DOI: 10.1016/0149-7634(94)90051-5

[39] Shepard JD, Barron KW, Myers DA. Corticosterone delivery to the amygdala increases corticotropin-releasing factor mRNA in the central amygdaloid nucleus and anxiety-like behavior. Brain Research. 2000;**861**:288-295. DOI: 10.1016/s0006-8993(00)02019-9

[40] Koob GF, Le Moal M. Drug addiction, dysregulation of reward, and allostasis. Neuropsychopharmacology. 2001;**24**:97-129. DOI: 10.1016/S0893-133X(00)00195-0

[41] Koob GF, Bloom FE. Cellular and molecular mechanisms of drug dependence. Science. 1988;**242**:715-723. DOI: 10.1126/science.2903550

[42] Sterling P, Eyer J. Allostasis: A new paradigm to explain arousal pathology. In: Fisher S, Reason J, editors. Handbook

of Life Stress, Cognition and Health. Chichester: John Wiley; 1988. pp. 629-649

[43] Koob GF. Brain stress systems in the amygdala in addiction. Brain Research. 2009;**1293**:61-75. DOI: 10.1016/j.brainres.2009.03.038

[44] Hennessy JW, Levine S. Stress, arousal, and the pituitary-adrenal system: A psychoendocrine hypothesis. In: Sprague JM, Epstein AN, editors. Progress in Psychobiology and Physiological Psychology. 8th ed. New York: Academic Press; 1979. pp. 133-178

[45] Pfaff D. Brain Arousal and Information Theory: Neural and Genetic Mechanisms. Cambridge, MA: Harvard University Press; 2006

[46] Rasmussen DD, Boldt BM, Bryant CA, Mitton DR, Larsen SA, Wilkinson CW. Chronic daily ethanol and withdrawal: 1. Long-term changes in the hypothalamo-pituitary-adrenal axis. Alcoholism, Clinical and Experimental Research. 2000;**24**:1836-1849. DOI: 10.1016/j.alcohol.2006.06.007

[47] Goeders NE. Stress and cocaine addiction. The Journal of Pharmacology and Experimental Therapeutics. 2002;**301**:785-789. DOI: 10.1124/jpet.301.3.785

[48] Sharp BM, Matta SG. Detection by in vivo microdialysis of nicotine-induced norepinephrine secretion from the hypothalamic paraventricular nucleus of freely moving rats: Dose-dependency and desensitization. Endocrinology. 1993;**133**:11-19. DOI: 10.1007/978-3-0348-7445-8_20

[49] Semba J, Wakuta M, Maeda J, Suhara T. Nicotine withdrawal induces subsensitivity of hypothalamic-pituitary-adrenal axis to stress in rats: Implications for precipitation of depression during smoking cessation. Psychoneuroendocrinology. 2004;**29**:215-226. DOI: 10.1016/s0306-4530(03)00024-6

[50] Alheid GF, Heimer L. New perspectives in basal forebrain organization of special relevance for neuropsychiatric disorders: The striatopallidal, amygdaloid, and corticopetal components of substantia innominata. Neuroscience. 1988;**27**:1-39. DOI: 10.1016/0306-4522(88)90217-5

[51] Johnston JB. Further contributions to the study of the evolution of the forebrain. Journal of Comparative Neurology. 1923;**35**:337-481. DOI: 10.1002/cne.900350502

[52] Heimer L, Alheid G. Piecing together the puzzle of basal forebrain anatomy. In: Napier TC, Kalivas PW, Hanin I, editors. The Basal Forebrain: Anatomy to Function. Advances in Experimental Medicine and Biology. Vol. 295. New York: Plenum Press; 1991. pp. 1-42

[53] Selye H. A syndrome produced by diverse nocuous agents. The Journal of Neuropsychiatry and Clinical Neurosciences. 1998;**10**:230-231

[54] Reul JM, de Kloet ER. Two receptor systems for corticosterone in rat brain: Microdistribution and differential occupation. Endocrinology. 1985;**117**:2505-2511

[55] Fuchs E, Czeh B, Kole MH, Michaelis T, Lucassen PJ. Alterations of neuroplasticity in depression: The hippocampus and beyond. European Neuropsychopharmacology. 2004;**14**(Suppl 5):S481-S490

[56] Swaab DF, Bao AM, Lucassen PJ. The stress system in the human brain in depression and neurodegeneration. Ageing Research Reviews. 2005;**4**:141-194

[57] Rasmuson S, Nasman B, Carlstrom K, Olsson T. Increased levels

of adrenocortical and gonadal hormones in mild to moderate Alzheimer's disease. Dementia and Geriatric Cognitive Disorders. 2002;**13**:74-79

[58] Giubilei F, Patacchioli FR, Antonini G, Sepe Monti M, Tisei P, Bastianello S, et al. Altered circadian cortisol secretion in Alzheimer's disease: Clinical and neuroradiological aspects. Journal of Neuroscience Research. 2001;**66**:262-265

[59] Sapolsky RM. Glucocorticoid toxicity in the hippocampus: Temporal aspects of neuronal vulnerability. Brain Research. 1985;**359**:300-305

[60] Belanoff JK, Rothschild AJ, Cassidy F, DeBattista C, Baulieu EE, Schold C, et al. An open label trial of C-1073 (mifepristone) for psychotic major depression. Biological Psychiatry. 2002;**52**:386-392

[61] Sapolsky RM, Krey LC, McEwen BS. The neuroendocrinology of stress and aging: The glucocorticoid cascade hypothesis. Endocrine Reviews. 1986;**7**:284-301

Chapter 3

Biomarkers of Diseases: Their Role in Emergency Medicine

Anoop T. Chakrapani

Abstract

Biomarkers have been playing an increasingly significant role in clinical decision making processes worldwide. Numerous studies are being undertaken across the globe in the elusive search for the ideal biomarker for each clinical condition. In the emergency department, where rapid diagnosis of various diseases like acute coronary syndromes, pulmonary embolism, heart failure, sepsis, acute renal failure etc. is of utmost importance, specific biomarkers can expedite the time to diagnosis and treatment. To enumerate, the following biomarkers have proved their worth within the setting of emergency departments across the world. The role of cardiac troponins and CK-MB has been well established in the clinical algorithms to detect myocardial infarction. Newer markers like Heart Fatty Acid Binding Protein (H-FABP), BNP, Pro BNP as well as Ischemia modified albumin (IMA) are coming into the fray in the detection of cardiovascular emergencies, especially in the detection of heart failure. Novel biomarkers like Mid-region Proadrenomedullin (MR-proADM) are found to be useful in sepsis along with Tumour necrosis factor-alpha (TNF-alpha), Interleukins and Presepsin in burns patients. Human neutrophil gelatinase-associated lipocalin (NGAL) levels can detect renal failure much earlier than conventional methods. S100 calcium binding protein B (S100B) has been found to be useful in detection of CNS injury and hence can be used to avoid unnecessary radiation to patients in the form of CT scans. Point of care testing of many of these biomarkers in the Emergency department itself paves way for a revolutionary step in faster emergency care delivery and better patient outcomes.

Keywords: biomarker, emergency medicine, troponin, sepsis, burns, acute kidney injury, head injury

1. Introduction

According to the National Institute of Health (NIH) Biomarkers Working Group, a biological marker (biomarker) is defined as "a characteristic that is objectively measured and evaluated as an indicator of normal biological processes, pathogenic processes, or pharmacologic responses to a therapeutic intervention" [1].

Worldwide, biomarkers have been primarily studied specifically in the setting of diseases. Even so, it is imperative to understand the concept that a biomarker in the human milieu can be present as a result of normal physiological functioning and need not be the result of a pathological process always. Analysis of various biomarkers, both quantitatively and qualitatively have resulted in better understanding of physiological as well as pathological processes of the human body. An ideal biomarker should aid in early diagnosis, help in risk stratification, be able to monitor response to treatment modalities and predict outcomes better than the clinical processes and investigations existing in medical practice at that point of time [2].

In medical practice, biomarkers can be of diagnostic or prognostic value. In the setting of practicing Emergency medicine, diagnostic biomarkers assume greater significance. In the Emergency department, where time is of the essence, diagnostic biomarkers help in quick clinical decision making as well as patient disposition. A biomarker that is able to make a clinical differentiation between two similar disease conditions is highly valuable for an emergency physician. This helps in rapid diagnosis, which leads to faster treatment initiation. Faster the treatment can be initiated, faster the patient movement. A faster TAT (turnaround time) for patients in the ED translates to lesser waiting times in the ED. An ideal biomarker in the Emergency department should have the following characteristics—High diagnostic accuracy which involves a high degree of sensitivity with reasonable specificity, should be reproducible across platforms and should be cost effective to the patient and the clinician.

Numerous biomarkers have been extensively studied for the purpose of clinical utility, but only a few handfuls have proved their mettle in clinical practice. The abundance of biomarker tests available, pose a not so friendly dilemma to the clinician of the present. Understandably, there is still a long way to traverse from the laboratory table to the patient bedside. Numerous trials and research activities are underway across the world in the field of biomarkers. Most of them are still in various phases of preclinical trials and are expected to be available by the patient's bedside in a few years' time.

In modern clinical practice, biomarkers are being used more and more for clinical decision making. The current gamut of biomarkers available in the clinical realm have changed the way we practice medicine. The increase in the use of biomarkers for clinical decision making has expedited the patient disposition to a great extent. Having said that, there is also the other side of the coin which is the increase in the health care cost. The over dependence of clinicians on biomarkers should be viewed with caution as this escalates the overall cost of treatment and the patients will have to bear that burden. The decision to make use of biomarkers in the clinical context should be individualised and targeted to prevent its overuse or abuse [3]. This will put a strain on the already scarce resources in the health care sector. It is always pertinent to remember that—A biomarker should always be evaluated in the clinical context and should never be used as a standalone tool for clinical decision making.

In Emergency medical practice, majority of the biomarker work has been focussed in the field of cardiology, renal failure and sepsis, as early detection and prompt interventions in the early phases of the diseases can significantly alter the natural course of the disease and improve the patient morbidity and mortality. Other areas of focus are hepatic diseases, traumatic brain injury, venous thromboembolism etc., where biomarkers are increasingly being tested for their clinical utility. Therefore, the chapter focuses in detail on these clinically significant biomarkers.

2. Acute coronary syndromes

Acute coronary syndromes have been in the forefront of novel biomarker evaluation research due to its widespread prevalence as well as the need for detection in a time sensitive manner. Almost 20 million patients with symptoms of acute coronary syndromes present to emergency departments in North America and Europe annually [4, 5]. Numerous studies have been performed on various biomarkers, the conventional markers as well as high sensitive variants, and also with respect to different time frames. In the Emergency department, making a rapid diagnosis of acute myocardial infarction is of utmost importance, as *'time is muscle'*. The earlier a diagnosis of ACS can be made, the earlier revascularisation can be initiated. Early treatment can decrease the morbidity and mortality to a significant extent in case of ACS. At the same time, it is also important to make sure deserving patients are disposed of from the ED as soon as possible in a time dependent manner once ACS is ruled out. This assumes more significance in EDs that receive a high volume of patients and need patients to be either admitted for further workup or discharged in a timely manner. At the same time, discharging patients from the ED always has a risk of patients ending up in an adverse cardiac event. Institutional protocols that include serial biomarker evaluation help in minimising these risks to a great extent.

Historically, biomarkers like LDH (lactate dehydrogenase) and AST (aspartate aminotransferase) were tried in the detection of an acute coronary syndrome especially towards the end of 20th century. Their clinical significance slowly began to decline with the advent of better alternatives as well as lack of specificity. The next in line were the markers with better specificity and sensitivity, namely—the troponins and creatine kinase. As the 21st century is taking its foothold, the scientific community is focussing its attention on these biomarkers for detection of acute coronary events, a leading cause of death worldwide. The research was primarily focussed on Creatine Kinase – MB fraction, which used to be the gold standard of evaluation of ACS. But, that has given way to the newer biomarkers—Troponin I and Troponin T – both conventional and high sensitive, which are being studied extensively across the globe.

2.1 Creatine kinase: MB

Creatine Kinase is an intracellular enzyme with a dimeric molecule which has 3 isoforms—CK-MM (muscle), CK-BB (brain) and CK-MB (myocardium), based on the organ of origin. CK-MB is the isoenzyme fraction which is predominantly seen in cardiac muscle and hence the utility in detecting cardiac muscle damage. This marker is leaked into the systemic circulation from the cellular cytosol due to disruption of the cell membrane as a result of myocardial injury. This marker can be assayed by a clinician to help in the diagnosis of myocardial infarction. CK-MB isoenzyme can be detected in the bloodstream about 4–6 hours after the onset of chest pain. It peaks by 12–24 hrs and returns to baseline by 12–48 hours. This short time window of rise and fall of CK MB is especially useful in detecting reinfarction or infarct extension in a patient in whom the troponin values might be already elevated as a result of an infarct. It is also helpful in identifying complications in patients who have undergone revascularization procedures in the cardiac care unit. The reference values for CK-MB are as follows—males: $\leq$ 7.7 ng/mL and females: $\leq$ 4.3 ng/mL. CK MB assay should always be viewed with a pinch of salt since it is a subunit of the total CK in the system. Abnormal elevations of CK MB can be detected along with an increased level of total CK in cases of traumatic muscle injuries, rhabdomyolysis, myopathies etc. It is worthwhile to note that the normally CK-MB fraction accounts for only 3–5% of the total CK in the body and any increase beyond 30–50% of the total CK should prompt suspicion of abnormal beta subunit synthesis. But, over the past few years, the burden of diagnosis of acute myocardial injury has been shifted on to the shoulders of troponins [6].

2.2 Cardiac troponins

Troponin is a complex protein molecule comprising of three regulatory proteins playing an integral role in the contraction of cardiac and skeletal muscle. These three subunits are namely—Troponin I (TnI), Troponin T (TnT) and Troponin C (TnC). Each subunit has a unique function. Troponin T binds to the troponin components of Tropomyosin, troponin I inhibits the interaction of myosin with actin and troponin C has the sites for binding of calcium ions to initiate muscle contraction.

Similar to creatine kinase, any cellular injury leads to leakage of the troponins into the systemic circulation thereby providing a window for diagnosis of acute myocardial infarction. Troponins have much higher specificity and sensitivity than creatine kinase. The utility of cardiac troponins especially – Troponin T and Troponin I has been validated in various studies across the world and hence has been incorporated into the diagnostic guidelines of acute myocardial infarction.

Normally troponins are not detectable in the bloodstream due to the minute quantities in open circulation, which is <0.01 ng/mL for Troponin T and ≤ 0.04 ng/mL for Troponin I. After a myocardial injury, elevated troponin levels in the bloodstream can be detected within a period of 4–6 hours, by conventional methods. The reason for this delay in detection has been attributed to the molecular weight and size (21–37 kDa). This can cause clinically significant delay in the diagnosis of myocardial infarction especially in the setting of nonspecific ECG changes. This has led to the advent of high sensitive assays which can detect troponins at much lower levels (at the levels of ng/L) and that too, much earlier than conventional methods. Troponins can be detected as early as 2 hours after the ischemic event by high sensitive troponin assays currently in clinical practice. This also has a caveat, that is, troponin levels can be detected in the circulation even without myocardial injury [4, 5]. Hence a troponin value above the 99th percentile is taken as a diagnostic cut-off for detection of myocardial ischemia. A 20% rise or fall from the baseline within a period of 3–6 hours can confirm the diagnosis of an acute myocardial infarction according to the National Academy of Clinical Biochemistry [6]. It has been recommended by the American college of Cardiology (ACC) that serial values of troponin be considered at 6–9 hr. intervals to rule out NSTEMI [7]. European Society of Cardiology has also reiterated the importance of doing serial assessments of troponins rather than making a clinical decision based on a single value [8]. In a recent large multicentre evaluation in patients with suspected ACS who presented within 8 hours of symptom onset, it was found that it was possible to diagnose ACS with 3-hour marker samples rather than the conventional method of doing serial markers at 6 hour intervals, without losing out on the diagnostic accuracy [9]. Along with clinical evidence of MI, an elevation of troponin level more than 5 times the upper limit compared to the baseline is needed to diagnose a PCI-related MI and more than 10 times the upper limit to diagnose a CABG-related MI [10]. Multiple studies have shown that there is correlation between the levels of troponins and development of adverse cardiac events [11, 12].

Elevated troponin levels may not always indicate myocardial injury [13, 14]. It can also be elevated in non-ischemic conditions as well. A rise/fall in troponin levels are needed to detect acute MI in patients in whom troponins will be elevated otherwise, like renal failure. Even though sensitivity is increased, specificity has come down which may indicate an underlying disease than an acute coronary event. Various causes of nonischemic elevation of troponins are detailed in the below table (**Table 1**). The troponin levels have to be interpreted only in the appropriate clinical setting, failing which the physician may be misled to an alternate diagnosis [15].

2.3 Other contenders

Numerous other biomarkers have piqued the interest of the scientific community to identify acute coronary events more early as well as more precisely. Very few have actually stood on their own when compared to troponin studies. The most

Cardiac	Non Cardiac
• Congestive cardiac failure	• Pulmonary Embolism
• Myocarditis	• Renal failure
• Pericarditis	• Sepsis
• Infiltrative diseases	• Stroke
	• Blunt chest trauma

Table 1.
Examples of non ACS-causes of elevated troponin levels:

• Myoglobin (Mb) P
• Heart Fatty Acid Binding Protein (H-FABP)
• Glycogen Phosphorylase-BB (GP-BB)
• NT-Pro-Brain Natriuretic Peptide (NT-ProBNP)
• D-Dimer
• High Sensitivity C-Reactive Protein (HsCRP)
• Myeloperoxidase (MPO)
• Matrix Metalloproteinase-9 (MMP-9)
• Pregnancy Associated Plasma Protein-A (PAPP-A)
• Soluble CD40 Ligand (SCD40L)

Table 2.
Newer biomarkers for cardiac ischemia.

common drawback being the cost of the investigation as well as availability. Some of the examples are discussed below.

Myoglobin (Mb) peaks within minutes of cardiac ischemia. With the recent advancements for detection of hs-troponin levels, the utility of Mb has come down in the diagnostic algorithm [16]. A few examples of other novel biomarkers of myocardial ischemia/injury that have undergone clinical trials are given below in **Table 2**. They include cardiac intracellular proteins, markers of neurohormonal activation, markers for haemostatic activity, vascular inflammation markers etc. [17]. In this study, the assessment of H-FABP within the first 4 h of symptoms was found to be superior to cTnT for detection of MI. But the reduced specificity of H-FABP is presently limiting its usefulness in clinical practice. Soluble CD40 ligand and choline which are biomarkers signalling the instability of atherosclerotic plaque formation, have been studied, but did not show add any prognostic or diagnostic value to the existing ones in practice. But the other biomarkers they studied along with this, did not show any favourable clinical significance.

3. Cardiac failure

Cardiac failure is a complex process involving a multitude of pathophysiological processes. As a result of this, various biomarkers have been identified which correlate with specific aspects of heart failure. The marker which has made its mark in a clinically significant manner are the natriuretic peptides-B type natriuretic peptide (BNP) and NT pro BNP.

3.1 B type natriuretic peptide (BNP) & NT pro BNP

BNP is secreted from the ventricles as a result of neurohormonal activation due to volume overload and resultant stretching of the myocardial muscle fibres. In patients with left ventricular dysfunction/failure, high plasma levels of BNP and NT pro BNP are specific for elevated filling pressures in the cardiac chambers. This can be used in the clinical context for the diagnosis as well as prognostication of cardiac failure. ProBNP is a 108-amino acid polypeptide precursor which is stored in secretory granules in both ventricles and, to a lesser extent, in the atria. After proBNP is secreted, it is cleaved to the 76-peptide, biologically inert N-terminal fragment NT-proBNP and the 32-peptide, biologically active hormone BNP. BNP is rapidly cleared from the circulation; the plasma half-life being approximately 20 min. No receptor-mediated clearance of NT-proBNP is known to occur, because of which NT-proBNP has a prolonged half-life of 60–120 min. The reference values for NT-proBNP varies widely with age and gender, which can be tricky for the clinician while assessing patients, especially in the elderly population (**Table 3**).

In the multicentre Breathing Not Properly Study [18], using plasma BNP level of 100 pg/mL as cut off, gave a sensitivity of 90%, specificity of 76% and a diagnostic accuracy of 81% which was superior to clinical assessment alone in a series of 1586 patients who presented to the ED with acute dyspnoea. A BNP level < 100 pg/ml or an NT-proBNP level < 300 pg/ml can essentially rule out Acute HF in most cases. When using N-terminal proBNP for the diagnosis of acute CHF, a value of 900 pg/mL has high specificity and sensitivity.

Apart from left ventricular failure, these biomarkers can be elevated in numerous other conditions which can cause myocardial stretch. Patients with right ventricular failure secondary to pulmonary embolism or pulmonary hypertension, valvular heart disease, arrhythmias such as atrial fibrillation, renal failure and advanced age may also have elevated levels of BNP or NT-proBNP [19]. In severe renal failure, the NT-pro BNP value of >1200 pg/mL is needed to make a diagnosis of cardiac failure. A common clinical scenario in which the patient is obese, the pro-BNP values can be falsely lower which can mask cardiac failure and lead to misdiagnosis.

The European Society of Cardiology Task Force has recommended that the algorithm for HF diagnosis should include an NP assay as the first step along with electrocardiography (ECG) and chest X-ray [20]. Biomarkers are not just useful in the diagnostic algorithm, but also in guiding treatment. In a meta-analysis [21] of 2686 patients in 12 randomised trials, the researchers found that the use of cardiac peptides to guide pharmacologic therapy significantly reduces mortality and HF related hospitalisation in patients with chronic HF.

As discussed in the previous section, Troponin I (TnI) also plays an important role in the pathophysiological profile of cardiac failure. Newer markers that have potential to be significance in the future for diagnosis and prognosis in heart failure include high-sensitivity C-reactive protein (hsCRP), uric acid and

Age	Males	Females
≤45 yrs	10–51 pg/mL	10–140 pg/mL
45–70 yrs	10–100 pg/mL	10–206 pg/mL
≥70 yrs	10–138 pg/mL	10–1263 pg/mL

Table 3.
Reference values for NT-ProBNP:

myeloperoxidase (MPO), soluble toll-like receptor-2 (ST2) and soluble fms-like tyrosine kinase receptor-1 (sFlt-1). Recently, a study in which the amount of exhaled acetone is measured has shown promise as a newer non-invasive modality for cardiac failure assessment [22]. A recent study attempted to evaluate the predictive utility of these biomarkers with a multimarker score which included BNP, troponin I and creatinine apart from the above markers. They concluded that a multimarker score significantly improves prediction of adverse events in ambulatory patients with chronic heart failure [23]. But, NACB's practice guidelines on cardiac biomarker testing specifically recommends against routine use of biomarker testing only for risk stratification [24]. The newer entries into this field include galectin-3 [25], MR-proANP (midregion pro–atrial natriuretic peptide) [26], MR-proADM (mid regional pro-adrenomedullin), co-peptin, adiponectin, pentraxin-3, soluble ICAM-1(intercellular adhesion molecule-1), PAPP-A (pregnancy associated plasma protein A) etc.

4. Pulmonary embolism

In a case of suspected pulmonary embolism, laboratory evaluation by biomarker levels is primarily helpful in ruling out the diagnosis in low probability scenarios, rather than ruling in a confirmation of a diagnosis. D-dimer has been in clinical use extensively since the past few decades and the other markers which are increasingly used are troponins, BNP and Ischemia modified albumin (IMA).

4.1 D-dimer

D-dimer is a degradation product produced by plasmin during fibrinolysis. The reference value of D-dimer is ≤500 ng/mL Fibrinogen equivalent Units (FEU). It has very low specificity, but a high sensitivity. Due to the low specificity, a clinical diagnosis of pulmonary embolism requires a strong clinical suspicion. In order to help the clinician in this regard, various scoring systems to assess the probability of making a diagnosis of PE have been devised. Well's criteria and its modified version are among the most commonly used. These scoring systems assist the clinician in assessing the probability of a diagnosis of PE along with the blood levels of the biomarker used. In patients with a low pretest probability of PE as assessed by well's criteria and a negative d-dimer value, the diagnosis of pulmonary embolism can be essentially ruled out without any probability of adverse events happening later [27, 28].

4.2 Ischemia modified albumin (IMA)

Ischemia modified albumin (IMA) is a newer marker that has shown potential as a substitute for D-dimer as it has been found to be better than the latter in a few studies due to its better positive predictive value [29]. The reference value for IMA is ≤0.540 ABSU. In patients with pulmonary embolism, more so in those who develop RV dysfunction, other biomarkers like troponins and BNP are also found to be elevated. This occurs due to the increased pulmonary vascular resistance, pulmonary artery pressure and resultant RV afterload. The elevated troponin levels can pose a dilemma for a clinician who wants to rule out ACS as well in the clinical setting as the symptoms of both the conditions may overlap significantly. The elevated levels of BNP/NT pro-BNP in patients with pulmonary embolism have been found to be associated with increase in risk for complications and 30-day mortality [30].

5. Sepsis

Sepsis is a complex process that stems from a combination of features of a systemic inflammatory response to a known or presumed infection. It is associated with a very high mortality rate around 30% not to mention the significant economic impact on the healthcare system [31]. Sepsis can be viewed as a chain of events in the body as a response to an inciting agent through an inflammatory pathway. This provides clinicians the opportunity to diagnose sepsis early by either picking up the inciting agent or the inflammatory response to the agent. More than 170 biomarkers have been identified as useful for evaluating sepsis [32], which itself points to the fact that none of them can be used as a single marker for accurate diagnosis or prognosis. C-reactive protein, procalcitonin and serum lactate are among the prominent ones used extensively worldwide at present.

5.1 C-reactive protein

C-Reactive protein, one of the most commonly used markers for sepsis, is synthesised in the liver as an acute phase reactant. The normal levels in a healthy adult individual tends to be below 10 mg/L. Depending on the severity, any stress or stimulus can cause an elevation in the CRP levels, even manifold up to 500 mg/L. The levels peak around 36–48 hrs and the plasma half-life is approx. 19 hrs. Although very commonly used as an inflammatory marker, it lacks specificity as it is found to be elevated in numerous conditions like post-operative patients, burns, myocardial infarction and inflammatory/rheumatic diseases as well [33]. It can be elevated even in normal individuals especially in elderly as well as pregnancy. Moreover, even a viral infection can cause a mild increase in the serum levels of CRP, contrary to popular belief. The sensitivity and specificity of CRP as a marker for bacterial infections are 68–92% and 40–67%, respectively [34, 35]. CRP plasma levels have shown to correlate with the severity of infection [36] which makes it a useful marker to assess the response to pharmacological treatment.

5.2 Procalcitonin (PCT)

It is a 116-amino acid polypeptide which is the prohormone of calcitonin. It has a short half-life (25–30 hours), and is encoded by the *CALC-1* gene. PCT is normally produced by neuroendocrine cells, mainly in the thyroid (C-cells), from which calcitonin is derived which is responsible for regulation of calcium metabolism in the body. It is also produced in low amounts in other neuroendocrine cells in the intestine and lungs. The *CALC-1* gene is normally suppressed in non-endocrine tissues. Bacterial infection stimulates *CALC-1*gene transcription in non-endocrine cells [37], leading to increased PCT production which can be detected in the circulation making it a marker for diagnosis of bacterial infection and sepsis. PCT is released from various organs including lung, liver, kidney, pancreas, spleen, colon, and even adipose tissues in infectious conditions. In healthy individuals, the serum PCT levels are <0.1 ng/ml, which increases in response to an infective stimulus. Serum PCT levels begin to rise around 4 hrs after the insult and peaks by 24 hrs. The half-life of PCT is approx. 24 hrs and after the infectious process has started resolving, PCT levels decrease by almost 50% every day [38]. In a systematic review and meta-analysis, PCT with a cut-off median value of 1.1 ng/mL was found to be more specific (specificity - 81%) than CRP (67%) for differentiating bacterial infection among hospitalised patients [39]. PCT also has a sensitivity of 77% which makes it a useful marker for early diagnosis of sepsis [40]. These features make PCT a favourable biomarker to be used for guidance of antibiotic stewardship as well to reduce the ever increasing inappropriate use/abuse of antibiotics [41].

5.3 Serum lactate

Lactate is produced in the body even normally, which gets cleared off rapidly in healthy individuals. But, in cases of sepsis and resultant hypoperfusion, the levels of lactic acid increase when anaerobic metabolism increases in the body. Lactate clearance has been shown in a prominent light in the 'Early goal directed therapy' of septic patients. This indicates that, more than a diagnostic marker, lactate has prognostic significance in patients with sepsis. Recent studies have shown that patients with even a milder increase in serum levels in the range of 2–4 mmol/L were at an increased risk of morbidity and mortality [42]. In a study conducted in an urban academic centre which included 1278 patients with infections, those with lactate levels above 4 mmol/L had higher in-hospital mortality rates than patients with lactate levels less than 2.5 mmol/L (28.4% vs. 4.9%) [43]. The bottom line is, the better the lactate clearance, better the outcome of the patient [44].

5.4 Proadrenomedullin (MR-proADM)

Adrenomedullin (ADM) is a 52-amino acid ringed peptide produced from endothelial cells in cardiovascular, renal, pulmonary, cerebrovascular and endocrine tissues. It is a potent endogenous vasodilator in the human body. ADM is not easily measurable due to its very short half-life of 22 minutes in the circulation, its rapid degradation by proteases, and the formation of complexes with circulating complement factor H [45]. The prohormone of ADM - ProADM can be used as a surrogate marker for this purpose as it is more easily quantifiable, and the tools required for this are available commercially. The mid-regional fragment of proadrenomedullin (MR-proADM) is a marker of endothelial dysfunction/inflammation and therefore can be seen in elevated levels in numerous disease conditions. Pro-ADM has been found to be an independent predictor for adverse outcomes in patients with COPD [46]. It has also been studied in the context of burns, in which it was found to have utility in early recognition of onset of sepsis in burns victims [47]. It is still early days for MR-proADM in routine clinical practice as many studies [48] have failed to demonstrate any added utility with respect to other less expensive parameters presently available. For healthy individuals, the reference values for MR pro ADM is <0.5 nmol/L.

5.5 Other markers of sepsis

Cytokines like TNF, IL-1β and IL-6 are the predominant inflammatory mediators responsible for the initial inflammatory response and the levels correlate with the organ damage and mortality [49]. Similarly, High-mobility group box 1 protein (HMGB1) and Macrophage migration inhibitory factor (MIF) are also found to increase in patients with severe sepsis and septic shock and is correlated with the degree of organ failure [50, 51]. Lipopolysaccharide-binding protein (LBS) is an acute phase protein which increases in sepsis and makes it useful as a diagnostic tool as well as a marker for severity of the disease [52, 53]. Other biomarkers like serum amyloid A, eosinophil count, mannan and antimannan, and IFN-γ-inducible protein 10 also show potential to be of use in the future.

6. Burns

In patients who are hospitalised with burns, sepsis is considered as one of the most important causes for mortality. Biomarkers which can help pick up the onset of sepsis in burn patients in the early phase itself will be useful in the proactive management of complications. Procalcitonin, Tumour necrosis factor-alpha (TNF-alpha), MR Pro-ADM, Interleukins 6, 8 & 10, Presepsin are among the major ones studied in this context in addition to assessment of single-nucleotide polymorphisms (SNPs) and leukocyte transcriptomes [54].

6.1 Procalcitonin

PCT has been extensively studied in the context of sepsis, but literature regarding studies in burns are much lesser in comparison to other critical conditions. Serum levels of PCT were found to be elevated in patients who developed infections after burns in one of the initial studies done in 1993 which had 9 burns patients included among the 79 general patients enrolled in the study [55]. In a recent meta-analysis of around 12 studies in burns patients led the investigators to believe that PCT has a strong ability to differentiate between patients with sepsis and without sepsis [56]. The study proposed that a PCT value >1.47 ng/mL can prompt the clinicians to initiate early antibiotic therapy to counter the development of sepsis and improve patient outcomes.

6.2 Tumour necrosis factor-alpha (TNF-alpha)

It is a proinflammatory cytokine and has been researched worldwide in various disease conditions among the host of numerous inflammatory mediators. It is produced ubiquitously in the body in response to various stimuli which can be infectious or ischemic in nature. They include endotoxins, complement system activation, hypoxia, ischemia as well as reperfusion [57]. TNF-alpha has been found to be elevated in burns and the values are seen to be higher in patients found to be in sepsis [58]. It has also been shown to have a prognostic value in burns victims. In burns patients who were treated with GM-CSF, the values of TNF alpha were shown to come down gradually as the treatment progressed [59], hence proving its role as a prognostic indicator. Reference value: ≤ 2.8 pg/mL.

6.3 Interleukins

The interleukins (ILs) are a large class of cytokines that promote cell-to-cell interactions and the stimulation of humoral or cell-mediated immune responses. They were initially thought to be produced only by the leukocytes, but have been found to be produced from numerous sources since then. The IL family consists of a huge number of members of which IL-6, IL-8 and IL-10 have been shown to be associated with evaluation of sepsis in burns patients. IL-6 has been found to be elevated in burns patients with sepsis [60]. It not only helps in the early diagnosis, but also has prognostic significance regarding the mortality as the levels have been found to be correlating with the size of the burns [61]. Recently, a meta-analysis of studies done on critically ill patients regarding markers of sepsis found IL-6 to have a high specificity, hence making it a suitable marker to confirm an infectious process [62]. Similarly, studies have found that IL-8 levels in burns patients correlate with the development of sepsis and multi-organ failure resulting in mortality [63]. The authors of the study opined that it can be used as a biomarker for monitoring the morbidity and mortality of burn patients developing sepsis. IL-10, similar to its counterparts, have been shown to have a correlation to development of sepsis in burn patients. Normally, the serum levels increase after the injury and decline later. But a failure to decline over time and being persistently elevated should point towards the development of an infective process and may increase the chances of mortality [64], hence making it a prognostic indicator in burn patients.

Some of the other notable markers pertaining to burns patients are - **Presepsin** which is the soluble form of cluster of differentiation 14 (CD14), a glycoprotein that functions as receptor for endotoxin complexes triggering signal transduction pathways implicated in systemic inflammation. In a study conducted on burns patients, Presepsin elevation preceded the elevation of CRP and PCT by 1 day as a marker of sepsis [65]. Several individual studies have reported the diagnostic accuracy of presepsin (sCD14-ST) for sepsis, but the results are inconsistent. Presepsin is an effective adjunct biomarker for the diagnosis of sepsis, but is insufficient to detect or rule out sepsis when used alone [66]. **Single-nucleotide polymorphisms (SNPs)** which are variations in a nucleotide at a specific chromosome location and has been linked to sepsis susceptibility and differences in prognosis in burns patients [67]. Gene-expression patterns like the **leukocyte transcriptome** shifts towards increased expression of genes involved in innate immunity and the inflammatory response and has been noted in burns patients [68]. But, most of these markers are not useful in day to day practice and have been limited to research settings at present. Nonetheless, the possibility of these markers making way into the clinical domain in the future cannot be ruled out.

7. Acute kidney injury

Conventionally, renal function tests which include serum levels of creatinine, urea and assessment of glomerular filtration rate are the methods used to quantify renal diseases. But, these conventional methods have a huge drawback. There is an unacceptable high time lag between the onset of tissue injury and derangement of these biochemical values. This hinders any active reno-protective interventions that may be initiated promptly. Moreover, the serum levels of these markers vary widely even in healthy individuals as it depends on various physical factors like age, gender, muscle mass etc. This has led the medical community to look for alternatives. Human neutrophil gelatinase-associated lipocalin (NGAL), kidney injury molecule 1 (KIM-1), interleukin-18 (IL-18), cystatin C, clusterin, fatty acid binding protein, and osteopontin are the prominent ones that have been studied and NGAL has been the most prominent one of the lot.

7.1 Neutrophil gelatinase-associated lipocalin (NGAL)

Neutrophil Gelatinase-associated Lipocalin (NGAL) is a protein that is expressed in neutrophils and has a role in innate immune response as well as repair and reepithelialisation in the kidney. In patients with acute kidney injury, ischemic or nonischemic type, plasma/urine levels of NGAL have been found to be elevated. (>50 μg/L) [69]. Both urinary and plasma levels of NGAL were found to increase by more than 10-fold within 2–6 hours of cardiac surgery in patients who later developed acute kidney injury. Urinary NGAL has been studied more extensively in paediatric population and has been found to be useful in detecting kidney injury following transplantation, cardiac surgery as well as contrast induced nephropathy early [70, 71].

Other markers that are being studied for their utility in kidney injury are Interleukin-18, Kidney injury molecule 1 (KIM-1), Cystatin – C, Sodium/Hydrogen Exchanger Isoform 3(NHE3) and Liver-type fatty acid binding protein (L-FABP). Kidney injury molecule 1 (KIM-1) and Interleukin-18 are found to be elevated in case of ischemic Acute Tubular Necrosis [72, 73]. Cystatin-C has been found to be better at estimating the GFR than the conventional method using creatinine [74]. Sodium/Hydrogen Exchanger Isoform 3(NHE3), which is found in the urine following tubular injury, has been found to be better than fractional excretion of sodium in differentiating between pre renal and intrinsic renal causes for renal failure [75]. Liver-type fatty acid binding protein (L-FABP) has also shown promise in animal studies for early detection of AKI and is being adapted as a possible biomarker for AKI [76].

8. Traumatic brain injury

8.1 Traumatic brain injury—acute injury

Traumatic brain injury is a major cause of morbidity and mortality across the world [77]. The reasons are several, but the lion's share of the incidents can be attributed to the high speed motor vehicle collisions. In addition to that, there are other contributing factors like falls as well as injuries due to contact sports. The acute injuries can be devastating and even fatal, but a huge number of those patients also develop chronic neurological sequelae which can be debilitating [78]. Given the complexity of the situation, the understanding of the mechanisms and pathophysiology of these chronic conditions are much less understood compared to their acute counterparts [79].

Traumatic Brain Injury (TBI) can be classified into acute or chronic based on the acuity of the event. Acute traumatic events as a result of MVA (motor vehicle accidents), falls or sporting events mostly result in immediate clinical symptoms or signs that are often diagnosed with the help of neuroimaging immediately by the clinician. A concussion as a result of contact sports or accidents can result in clinical features which can range from mild dizziness to complete unconsciousness. But, it will exhibit no discernible defects in neuroimaging of the patient [80]. Therefore it becomes a clinical diagnosis rather than a radiological diagnosis. Many patients, especially sportspersons who are part of contact sports like boxing have exhibited persistent symptoms for hours to days to months after the insult [81]. The shearing forces in an acceleration/deceleration injury causes axonal damage which is often responsible for the clinical manifestations. The acute event leads to a primary insult to the central nervous system which can manifest as cerebral oedema or even intracranial haemorrhage. This in turn leads to increase in the intracranial pressure which in turn causes cerebral hypoperfusion and resultant tissue hypoxia [82].

Traumatic head injury is not an area which usually requires a biomarker evaluation from the Neurosurgeon's point of view for the purpose of acute care. Clinical decision making is often dependent on neuroimaging, which is a CT scan usually. But, recently, the role of biomarkers has become important in the decision making process of getting a neuroimaging. This is done with a view of reducing the radiation exposure to patients with mild head injury. These biomarkers are not usually present in the circulation and their presence generally indicates a breach of Blood–brain barrier. Some of the important biomarkers described in the recent literature are Glial fibrillary acidic protein (GFAP), calcium binding protein S100B, and tau protein [83]. The most important one in the horizon is S100 calcium binding protein B (S100B), which is a glial-specific protein which is primarily expressed by a subtype of mature astrocytes. It is elevated in neuronal damage which makes it a potential marker for CNS insults. In a study done on 512 adult patients with mild head injury (GCS 14–15, loss of consciousness and/or amnesia and no additional risk factors), the researchers used protein S100B levels as a clinical tool to determine whether the patient needed a CT scan [84]. They found that adult patients with mild head injury, without additional risk factors and with S100B levels of <0.10 mcg/L within 3 hours of injury, can safely be discharged from the hospital without neuroimaging. A recent study done in Sweden tries to shed light on the utility of biomarkers like total tau, protein S100B and neuron-specific enolase in assessing concussion injuries in sports persons [85].

8.2 Traumatic brain injury - chronic Sequelae

Once the primary insult is over, the brain can suffer from secondary injury as a result of sequelae from the initial insult. This can occur after days, weeks, months or years after the initial event. This results from biochemical cascades that are triggered by the primary event. These secondary events are mediated by free radicals and reactive oxygen species that are generated as a result of tissue hypoxia, reperfusion injury and neuroinflammation [86]. The change in membrane permeability which results from the initial injury causes increase in the calcium uptake or activation of NMDA and AMPA receptors by glutamate can cause mitochondrial dysfunction [87]. Thus the inflammatory response leads to further cellular disruption and the vicious cycle continues to damage the nervous homeostasis. These inflammatory insults in the nervous system give rise to various inflammatory markers which can be detected in the system. These biomarkers have been extensively studied and their usefulness in the clinical environment hotly debated. Even though many of these markers many of them show enough promise within the confines of the laboratory, they are yet to come to the bedside to be used by the clinician in daily practice.

Many animal studies have demonstrated an increase in biochemical markers even after a single day after the insult and these can persist even after a month [88]. Acrolein, a post-traumatic neurotoxin can be quantified in brain tissue and can be elevated depending on the insult. A sustained upregulation has been demonstrated after brain injury, which suggests that it is a potential marker for neuronal injury and inflammation [89].

Proton Magnetic Resonance Spectroscopy (1H-MRS) is a technique which is able to measure the neurochemicals in the nervous system. This helps in detecting the neurotransmitters and metabolites, thereby quantifying the markers in various clinical conditions. Using this method, animal studies have found that endogenous antioxidants glutathione and ascorbic acid may be decreased up to 2 weeks follow ing the insult [90]. F2-isoprostane, a lipid peroxidation by-product, has been found to be elevated on chronic brain injury or Chronic Traumatic Encephalopathy (CTE) which manifests years after the insult(s).

As detected by Proton Magnetic Resonance Spectroscopy (^{1}H-MRS), there have been consistent results in detection of the following neurotransmitters in children with Autism Spectrum Disorder(ASD). There has been reduced levels of N-acetylaspartate (NAA), Creatine and phosphocreatine (Cr + PCr), Glutamine, Myo-Inositol and Choline containing compounds in the subcortical areas as well as cortical white matter and grey matter in varying degrees in children with ASD [91].

8.3 Neurodegenerative diseases

Neurodegenerative diseases can be extremely debilitating and distressing to not only the patient, but also the caregivers. Once diagnosed, the pathophysiological mechanisms can seldom be reversed and hence it becomes the source of social, financial and economic drain for not only families, but for the governmental health machinery itself. The social impact is huge, but the economic impact of these conditions cannot be ignored by any means.

Hence, it becomes imperative that the diagnosis can be made as early as possible thereby mitigating the scenario. An earlier diagnosis will help the clinician as well as the caregivers to come to a plan for further care of the patient. It is also essential to look at the therapeutic interventions which can arrest or at least slow down the progression of the disease. This is where the role of biomarkers come into picture. A biomarker can help in diagnosing a particular condition early. Even if the diagnosis cannot be confirmed, at least the possibility of the condition can be ascertained and hence be prepared against. This is where a biomarker helps in fighting the diseases which for all practical purposes, have no definitive curative measures available by the bedside.

Biomarkers in neurodegenerative conditions can be classified as fluid and radiological markers. Since radiology is an integral and essential part of assessment of the neurological system in modern medicine, many techniques have been developed which can detect the presence of markers within the brain tissue which can point towards the presence or likelihood of a particular disease condition. On the other hand, there are fluid biomarkers that can be detected in the fluid that flows all over the brain - the cerebrospinal fluid (CSF). Before we look into those markers, it needs to be kept in mind that quite a few markers have gone to the lab in the hunt for that perfect biomarker. But, none of them has been successful enough to be brought to the bedside for daily clinical practice. Among the many neurodegenerative conditions, Alzheimer's disease has been the most extensively studied, because of its prevalence and impact on the society. But the biomarkers used in Alzheimer's disease do overlap with many other conditions as well due to similarities in pathophysiology.

Biomarkers in neurodegenerative conditions can be detected in blood and cerebrospinal fluid (CSF) and are clubbed together to be called as fluid markers. The predominant ones are Amyloid β peptides/oligomers and Tau peptides. Neurofilament light chain (NfL), which is found in myelinated axons, is an important marker which indicates white matter damage and points towards neurodegeneration [92]. Serial NFL sampling in patients at risk of developing Alzheimer's Disease, can be used to predict brain atrophy rates, cognitive impairment and disease progression [93]. These can be estimated by assays in blood as well as CSF. The major disadvantage these markers face is the low specificity and that hinders its utility in clinical practice. Another set of markers or radiological distinction characteristics can be detected in MRI and PET scans and are termed as radiological biomarkers. MRI utilises the various imaging modalities available to detect white matter lesions that are present in many of the neurodegenerative diseases. These include reduction in the volume, thickness, presence of microbleeds, myelin, iron, neuromelanin within the brain tissue in specific regions. PET targets various Tau lesions and Amyloid β aggregates in various regions within the neuronal system to detect the possibility of neurodegeneration. Apart from these, there are genetic biomarkers or specific genes that can predict the possibility of a neurodegenerative disease condition (**Table 4**).

Gene(s)	Disease syndrome associated
APP, PSEN1, PSEN2	Familial - Early-onset Alzheimer's disease
ApoE (ε4 allele), TREM2	AD- Risk factors
MAPT, C9orf72, GRN	Behavioural-variant frontotemporal dementia
VCP, TARDBP, SOD1, FUS	Amyotrophic Lateral Sclerosis
HTT	Huntington's disease
SNCA, GBA	Parkinson's disease
PRNP	Prion Disease

Table 4.
Genetic biomarkers for neurodegenerative diseases.

8.3.1 Alzheimer's disease

It is a proteinopathy which is characterised by accumulation of Tau neurofibrillary tangles and extracellular Amyloid β plaques. These can be assessed by radiological methods as well as by looking at the fluid biomarkers. It has a prolonged pre-clinical phase where there Tau lesions can be found in the subcortical regions even before profound clinical symptoms appear [94]. Similarly amyloid β aggregates are initially found in the neocortical regions and later subcortical and cerebellar regions [95]. Plasma levels of Aβ42 has been found to be decreased compared to controls in a study [96]. The National Institute on Ageing and Alzheimer's Association Research Framework has defined AD by its underlying pathologic processes that can be documented by post-mortem examination or in vivo by biomarkers [97]. The biomarkers are classified into the 3 major groups- β amyloid deposition, pathologic tau, and neurodegeneration - AT(N). As and when newer biomarkers are discovered, they may be added into these categories. When it comes to therapeutics targeted based on these markers, there is still a long way to go to get these implemented in clinical practice. This may be due to the lack of direct correlation between the marker load with the clinical deterioration [98] as well as lack of specificity [99].

8.3.2 Parkinson's disease

It is the most common presentation of synucleinopathy. The presentation can be similar to other similar conditions like Dementia with Lewy bodies. The typical feature can be aggregation of α-synuclein in the form of Lewy bodies which starts in the subcortical regions and later spread into the other regions [100]. Apart from the mutations in the genes, causality has been attributed to pesticide exposure as well as traumatic brain injury [101].

8.3.3 Frontotemporal lobar degeneration

This encompasses a spectrum of disease conditions characterised by vacuolation, gliosis and neuronal loss in the cortical regions of the frontal and temporal lobes. Features of Tau protein accumulation, TDP-43 or fused in sarcoma can be seen in this condition [102]. Since they share a similar pathophysiology, Amyotrophic lateral sclerosis (ALS) and other similar motor neuron diseases are considered to be part of the same spectrum.

Huntington's disease is characterised by progressive neuronal loss and astrogliosis in the striatum along with prominent degeneration of the other cortical regions [103]. Similar to other disease conditions, there is limited data available to look at the therapeutic use of markers in HD also. Plasma levels of IL-8, TNF-α [104], and NfL may become useful in the coming years in this regard. A decrease in the uptake of phosphodiesterase-10 PET tracer in the strial region may become an important marker with regard to therapeutics in HD [105]. Diagnosis of Prion diseases like sporadic Creutzfeldt-Jakob disease (sCJD) is done by EEG, MRI or CSF based biomarkers with the use of real-time quaking-induced conversion (RT-QuIC) which is preferred over 14-3-3 protein detection [106].

Since many of the neurodegenerative conditions present late in clinical practice, it is imperative that in order to tackle this menace, the scientific community will have to bring forth tools that can detect these early as well us much ahead of the phase of clinical presentation, even decades. It is in this regard, the biomarkers have a major role to play, whether they are radiological or fluid markers. Genetic markers are useful when we are dealing with hereditary conditions or familial variants of neurodegenerative conditions. Confirmation of the diagnosis is essential in determining the treatment and initiating it at the earliest for the best possible response.

8.4 Newer modalities in the horizon

Even though the field of biomarker evaluation is not very old, it is a fast changing world and newer techniques are being added to the mix quite often. A recent technique is the Multimer Detection System-Oligomeric Aβ, which looks at the tendency of plasma proteins to oligomerize [107]. Immune-infrared sensor assay to measure blood vessels for the propensity of the amyloid protein to form β-sheets has also been tried with some success as a potential biomarker [108]. Measurement of locus coeruleus, an early affected region, using special MRI techniques is also being explored as a potential target [109].

9. Point of care tests (POCT)

POCT refers to diagnostic evaluation at or near the site of patient care. A POC lab is not within the institutional central laboratory, but nearer to the patient care setting like ED or ICU. POC testing of biomarkers is increasingly becoming the norm at the moment. This has been touted as the next revolutionary step in faster healthcare delivery in the Emergency department. But, the challenge lies in transferring the resultant advantage to improvement in patient care and disposition. The benefit demonstrated on paper should be translated to better patient care by the bedside. If the results of the POC testing do not alter the course of management of the patient, it defeats the whole purpose of POCT.

10. Future of biomarker use in emergency medicine

Biomarkers are being increasingly used in the Emergency departments for faster patient disposition. Recently efforts are being undertaken to include an array of biomarkers in the triage scoring itself as a method of risk stratification of patients presenting to the ED [110]. In this study, the researchers included biomarkers from 3 distinct biological pathways for risk stratification of general medical patients presenting to the ED. The study included biomarkers of inflammation (pro-adrenomedullin [ProADM]), stress (copeptin) and infection (procalcitonin). They used a multi-marker approach to stratify patients and came to a conclusion that all the markers strongly predicted the risk of death, ICU admission and high initial triage priority, especially ProADM. It is a possibility that these methods may get introduced in clinical practice in the not so distant future.

11. Conclusion

Biomarkers are among the best tools in the hand of the clinicians at present. Each and every clinical condition has been tagged with a quantifiable biomarker which helps in faster clinical diagnosis as well as prognostication. Overall this would lead towards better healthcare delivery to the patient. But, the sheer vast numbers and volumes of various biomarkers in the research pipeline points towards a glaring fact. There is no single marker that can give a complete picture of the patient's clinical condition. There is no ideal biomarker. A scoring system based on multiple markers would give a better picture than a single one. This accuracy always comes at a higher cost, which translates to more expensive healthcare delivery. There is dire requirement for better clinical validation among the various contenders in each disease process A biomarker based evaluation system, though more accurate, may not suit each and every healthcare facility, but needs to be tailored based on the adaptability and cost effectiveness suited to the society it caters to. Given the vast array of biomarker assays, clinicians should keep in mind that these should always be used as tools that compliment your clinical decision making process rather than replacing the process itself.

Acknowledgements

I would like to acknowledge the role of my wife, Aparna, who has been a pillar of support throughout the writing of this chapter just like she has been throughout our life together. I would also like to acknowledge the support given by my parents, friends as well as colleagues in my department, who made me what I am.

Conflict of interest

I have no conflict of interest to declare.

Abbreviations

ACC	American College of Cardiology
ACS	Acute Coronary Syndrome
AST	Aspartate aminotransferase
BNP	B type natriuretic peptide
CABG	Coronary Artery Bypass Grafting
CHF	Congestive Heart Failure
CNS	Central Nervous System
COPD	Chronic Obstructive Pulmonary Disease
CT	Computed Tomography
ECG	Electrocardiogram
ED	Emergency Department
H-FABP	Heart Fatty Acid Binding Protein
ICU	Intensive Care Unit
IL	Interleukin
IMA	Ischemia modified albumin
LDH	Lactate dehydrogenase
LVF	Left Ventricular Failure
MI	Myocardial Infarction
MR-proADM	Mid-regional Proadrenomedullin
NACB	National Academy of Clinical Biochemistry
NGAL	Neutrophil gelatinase-associated lipocalin
NSTEMI	Non ST Elevation Myocardial Infarction
NT pro BNP	N-Terminal pro B type natriuretic peptide
PCI	Percutaneous Coronary Intervention
POCT	Point of Care Testing
QC	Quality Control

STEMI	ST Elevation Myocardial Infarction
TNF	Tumour Necrosis Factor
TNF-alpha	Tumour necrosis factor-alpha

Author details

Anoop T. Chakrapani
Frimley Park Hospital, Frimley, United Kingdom

*Address all correspondence to: dranooptc@gmail.com

References

[1] Biomarkers Definitions Working Group. Biomarkers and surrogate endpoints: Preferred definitions and conceptual framework. Clinical Pharmacology and Therapeutics. 2001;**69**(3):89-95

[2] Chakrapani AT. Biomarkers in emergency medicine. In: David S, editor. Clinical Pathways in Emergency Medicine. New Delhi: Springer; 2016. DOI: https://doi.org/10.1007/978-81-322-2710-6_32

[3] Schuetz P, Aujesky D, Muller C, Muller B. Biomarker-guided personalised emergency medicine for all - hope for another hype? Swiss Medical Weekly. 2015;**145**:w14079

[4] Hollander JE, Than M, Mueller C. State-of-the-art evaluation of emergency department patients presenting with potential acute coronary syndromes. Circulation. *2016*;**134**:547-564. DOI: 10.1161/CirculationAHA.116.021886

[5] Saenger AK, Beyrau R, Braun S, Cooray R, Dolci A, Freidank H, et al. Multicentre analytical evaluation of a high-sensitivity troponin T assay. Clinica Chimica Acta. 2011 Apr 11;**412**(9-10):748-754

[6] Morrow DA, Cannon CP, Jesse RL, et al. National Academy of Clinical Biochemistry Laboratory medicine practice guidelines: Clinical characteristics and utilization of biochemical markers in acute coronary syndromes. Clinical Chemistry. 2007;**53**:552-574

[7] Anderson JL, Adams CD, Antman EM, Bridges CR, Califf RM, Casey DE Jr, et al. ACC/AHA 2007 guidelines for the management of patients with unstable angina/non-ST-Elevation myocardial infarction: a report of the American College of Cardiology/American Heart Association Task Force on Practice Guidelines. J Am Coll Cardiol. Aug 14 2007;**50**(7)

[8] Hamm CW, Bassand JP, Agewall S, Bax J, Boersma E, Bueno H, Caso P, Dudek D, Gielen S, Huber K, Ohman M, Petrie MC, Sonntag F, Uva MS, Storey RF, Wijns W, Zahger D: ESC Guidelines for the management of acute coronary syndromes in patients presenting without persistent ST-segment elevation: The Task Force for the management of acute coronary syndromes (ACS) in patients presenting without persistent ST-segment elevation of the European Society of Cardiology (ESC).ESC Committee for Practice Guidelines. Eur Heart J. 2011 Dec; 32(23):2999-3054.

[9] Diercks D.B, Peacock W.F, Hollander J.E, Singer A.J, Birkhahn R, Shapiro N: Diagnostic accuracy of a point-of-care troponin I assay for acute myocardial infarction within 3 hours after presentation in early presenters to the emergency department with chest pain. Am Heart J 2012;163:74-80.e4

[10] Thygesen K, Alpert JS, Jaffe AS, et al. Third universal definition of myocardial infarction. Journal of the American College of Cardiology. 2012;**60**:1581-1598

[11] Lindahl B, Toss H, Siegbahn A, Venge P, Wallentin L. Markers of myocardial damage and inflammation in relation to long-term mortality in unstable coronary artery disease. FRISC Study Group. Fragmin during Instability in Coronary Artery Disease. N Engl J Med. Oct 19 2000;343(16):1139-1147

[12] Newby LK, Christenson RH, OhmanEM,ArmstrongPW,ThompsonTD, Lee KL, et al. Value of serial troponin T measures for early and late risk stratification in patients with acute coronary syndromes. The GUSTO-IIa

Investigators. Circulation. Nov 3 1998;98(18):1853-1859

[13] Newby et al. ACCF 2012 Expert Consensus Document on Practical Clinical Considerations in the Interpretation of Troponin Elevations, A Report of the American College of Cardiology Foundation Task Force on Clinical Expert Consensus Documents. JACC Vol. 60, No. 23, December 11, 2012:2427-2463

[14] De Gennaro GL, Brunetti ND, Cuculo A, et al. Increased troponin levels in nonischemic cardiac conditions and noncardiac diseases. Journal of Interventional Cardiology. 2008;**21**:129-139

[15] Diamond GA, Kaul S. How would the reverend Bayes interpret high-sensitivity troponin? Circulation. 2010;**121**:1172-1175

[16] Eggers KM, Oldgren J, Nordenskjöld A, Lindahl B. Diagnostic value of serial measurement of cardiac markers in patients with chest pain: Limited value of adding myoglobin to troponin I for exclusion of myocardial infarction. American Heart Journal. Oct 2004;**148**(4):574-581

[17] Conor J. McCann Ben M. Glover Ian B.A. Menown Michael J. Moore Jane McEneny Colum G. Owens Bernie Smith Peter C. Sharpe Ian S. Young Jennifer A. Adgey; Novel biomarkers in early diagnosis of acute myocardial infarction compared with cardiac troponin T European Heart Journal, Volume 29, Issue 23, 1 December 2008, Pages 2843-2850,https://doi.org/10.1093/eurheartj/ehn363

[18] Maisel AS, Clopton P, Krishnaswamy P, Novak RM, McCord J, Hollander JE, et al. Impact of age, race, and sex on the ability of B-type natriuretic peptide to aid in the emergency diagnosis of heart failure: Results from the breathing not properly (BNP) multinational study. American Heart Journal. 2004;**147**(6):1078-1084

[19] Kim HN, Januzzi JL Jr. Natriuretic peptide testing in heart failure. Circulation. 2011;**123**:2015-2019

[20] Ray P, Delerme S, Jourdain P, Chenevier-Gobeaux C. Differential diagnosis of acute dyspnoea: the value of B natriuretic peptides in the emergency department. QJM. 2008;**101**:831-843

[21] Savarese G, Trimarco B, Dellegrottaglie S, Prastaro M, Gambardella F, Rengo G, et al. Natriuretic peptide-guided therapy in chronic Heart Failure: A meta-analysis of 2,686 patients in 12 randomized trials. PLoS One. 2013;**12**:e58287

[22] Marcondes-Braga FG, Gutz IGR, Batista GL, Saldiva PHN, Ayub-Ferreira SM, Issa VS, et al. Exhaled acetone as a new biomarker of heart failure severity. Chest. 2012 Aug;**142**(2):457-466

[23] Ky B, French B, Levy WC, et al. Multiple biomarkers for risk prediction in chronic heart failure. Circulation. Heart Failure. 2012;**5**:183-190

[24] Tang WH, Francis GS, Morrow DA, et al. National academy of clinical biochemistry laboratory medicine practice guidelines: Clinical utilization of cardiac biomarker testing in heart failure. Circulation. 2007;**116**:e99-e109

[25] De Boer RA, Yu L, van Veldhuisen DJ. Galectin-3 in cardiac remodelling and heart failure. Current Heart Failure Reports. 2010;7:1-8

[26] Maisel A, Mueller C, Nowak R, Peacock WF, Landsberg JW, Ponikowski P, Mockel M, Hogan C, Wu AH, Richards M, Clopton P, Filippatos GS, Di Somma S, Anand I, Ng L, Daniels LB, Neath SX, Christenson R, Potocki M, McCord J, Terracciano G, Kremastinos D, Hartmann O, von Haehling S,

Bergmann A, Morgenthaler NG, Anker SD. Mid-Region pro-hormone markers for diagnosis and prognosis in acute dyspnoea: results from the BACH (Biomarkers in acute heart failure) Trial, J Am Coll Cardiol , 2010, vol. 55 (pg. 2062-2076)

[27] Kearon C, Ginsberg JS, Douketis J, Turpie AG, Bates SM, Lee AY, et al. An evaluation of D-dimer in the diagnosis of pulmonary embolism: a randomized trial. Ann Intern Med. Jun 6 2006;144(11):812-821.

[28] Geersing GJ, Erkens PM, Lucassen WA, Büller HR, Cate HT, Hoes AW, et al. Safe exclusion of pulmonary embolism using the Wells rule and qualitative D-dimer testing in primary care: prospective cohort study. BMJ. Oct 4 2012;345:e6564

[29] Turedi S, Gunduz A, Mentese A, Topbas M, Karahan SC, Yeniocak S, et al. The value of ischemia-modified albumin compared with d-dimer in the diagnosis of pulmonary embolism. Respir Res. May 30 2008;9:49.

[30] Klok FA, Mos IC, Huisman MV. Brain-type natriuretic peptide levels in the prediction of adverse outcome in patients with pulmonary embolism: a systematic review and meta-analysis. Am J Respir Crit Care Med. Aug 15 2008;178(4):425-430

[31] Levy MM, Dellinger RP, Townsend SR, et al. The surviving sepsis campaign: results of an international guideline-based performance improvement program targeting severe sepsis. Intensive Care Medicine. 2010;**36**:222-231

[32] Pierrakos C, Vincent JL. Sepsis biomarkers: A review. Critical Care. 2010;**14**(1):R15

[33] Vincent JL, Donadello K, Schmit X. Biomarkers in the critically ill patient: C-reactive protein. Critical Care Clinics. 2011;**27**:241-251

[34] Simon L, Gauvin F, Amre DK, Saint-Louis P, Lacroix J. Serum procalcitonin and C-reactive protein levels as markers of bacterial infection: A systematic review and meta-analysis. Clinical Infectious Diseases. 2004;**39**:206-217

[35] Cho SY, Choi JH; Biomarkers of Sepsis; Infect Chemother. Mar 2014; 46(1): 1-12

[36] Póvoa P, Coelho L, Almeida E, Fernandes A, Mealha R, Moreira P, et al. C-reactive protein as a marker of infection in critically ill patients. Clinical Microbiology and Infection. 2005;**11**:101-108

[37] Becker KL, Nylen ES, White JC, Muller B, Snider RHJ. Procalcitonin and the calcitonin gene family of peptides in inflammation, infection, and sepsis: A journey from calcitonin back to its precursors. The Journal of Clinical Endocrinology and Metabolism. 2004;**89**(4):1512-1525

[38] Long B, Koyfman A. Ready for prime time? Biomarkers in sepsis. Emergency Medicine Clinics of North America. 2017;**35**(1):109 122

[39] Simon L, Gauvin F, Amre DK, Saint-Louis P, Lacroix J. Serum procalcitonin and C-reactive protein levels as markers of bacterial infection: A systematic review and meta-analysis. Clinical Infectious Diseases. 2004;**39**:206-217

[40] Wacker C, Prkno A, Brunkhorst FM, Schlattmann P. Procalcitonin as a diagnostic marker for sepsis: A systematic review and meta-analysis. The Lancet Infectious Diseases. 2013;**13**:426-435

[41] Kopterides P, Siempos II, Tsangaris I, Tsantes A, Armaganidis A. Procalcitonin-guided algorithms of antibiotic therapy in the intensive care unit: A systematic review

and meta-analysis of randomized controlled trials. Critical Care Medicine. 2010;**38**:2229-2241

[42] Mikkelsen ME, Miltiades AN, Gaieski DF, et al. Serum lactate is associated with mortality in severe sepsis independent of organ failure or shock. Critical Care Medicine. 2009;**37**:1670-1677

[43] Shapiro NI, Howell MD, Talmor D, Nathanson LA, Lisbon A, Wolfe RE, et al. Serum lactate as a predictor of mortality in emergency department patients with infection. Annals of Emergency Medicine. 2005;**45**:524-528

[44] Nguyen HB, Rivers EP, Knoblich BP, Jacobsen G, Muzzin A, Ressler JA, et al. Early lactate clearance is associated with improved outcome in severe sepsis and septic shock. Critical Care Medicine. 2004;**32**:1637-1642

[45] Lewis LK, Smith MW, Yandle TG, Richards AM, Nicholls MG. Adrenomedullin(1-52) measured in human plasma by radioimmunoassay: Plasma concentration, adsorption, and storage. Clinical Chemistry. 1998;**44**(3):571-577

[46] Maisel A, Mueller C, Nowak R, Peacock WF, Landsberg JW, Ponikowski P, et al. Mid-region pro-hormone markers for diagnosis and prognosis in acute dyspnea: results from the BACH (Biomarkers in Acute Heart Failure) trial. J Am Coll Cardiol. 2010 May 11;**55**(19):2062-2076

[47] Gille J, Ostermann H, Dragu A, Sablotzki A. MR-proADM: A new biomarker for early diagnosis of sepsis in burned patients. Journal of Burn Care & Research. 2017 Mar;**28**

[48] Gijs W.D. Landman, Peter R. van Dijk, Iefke Drion, Kornelis J.J. van Hateren, Joachim struck, Klaas H. Groenier, Rijk O.B. Gans, Henk J.G. Bilo, Stephan J.L. Bakker, NanneKleefstra; Midregional fragment of Proadrenomedullin, new-onset albuminuria, and cardiovascular and all-cause mortality in patients with type 2 diabetes (ZODIAC-30); Diabetes Care Mar 2014, 37 (3) 839-845

[49] Oberholzer A, Souza SM, Tschoeke SK, Oberholzer C, Abouhamze A, Pribble JP, et al. Plasma cytokine measurements augment prognostic scores as indicators of outcome in patients with severe sepsis. Shock. 2005 Jun;**23**(6):488-493

[50] Sundén-Cullberg J, Norrby-Teglund A, Rouhiainen A, Rauvala H, Herman G, Tracey KJ, et al. Persistent elevation of high mobility group box-1 protein (HMGB1) in patients with severe sepsis and septic shock. Critical Care Medicine. 2005 Mar;**33**(3):564-573

[51] Bozza FA, Gomes RN, Japiassú AM, Soares M, Castro-Faria-Neto HC, Bozza PT, et al. Macrophage migration inhibitory factor levels correlate with fatal outcome in sepsis. Shock. 2004;**22**:309-313

[52] Gaïni S, Koldkjaer OG, Pedersen C, Pedersen SS. Procalcitonin, lipopolysaccharide-binding protein, interleukin-6 and C-reactive protein in community-acquired infections and sepsis: A prospective study. Critical Care. 2006;**10**(2):R53

[53] Sakr Y, Burgett U, Nacul FE, Reinhart K, Brunkhorst F. Lipopolysaccharide binding protein in a surgical intensive care unit: A marker of sepsis? Critical Care Medicine. 2008 Jul;**36**(7):2014-2022

[54] Nunez Lopez O, Cambiaso-Daniel J, Branski LK, Norbury WB, Herndon DN. Predicting and managing sepsis in burn patients: Current perspectives. Therapeutics and Clinical Risk Management. 2017;**13**:1107-1117

[55] Assicot M, Gendrel D, Carsin H, Raymond J, Guilbaud J, Bohuon C. High

serum procalcitonin concentrations in patients with sepsis and infection. Lancet (London, England) 1993;341(8844):515-518

[56] Cabral L, Afreixo V, Almeida L, Paiva JA. The use of procalcitonin (PCT) for diagnosis of sepsis in burn patients: A meta-analysis. PLoS One. 2016;**11**(12):e0168475

[57] Parameswaran N, Patial S. Tumor necrosis factor-alpha signalling in macrophages. Critical Reviews in Eukaryotic Gene Expression. 2010;**20**(2):87-103

[58] Abdel-Hafez NM, Saleh Hassan Y, El-Metwally TH. A study on biomarkers, cytokines, and growth factors in children with burn injuries. Annals of Burns and Fire Disasters. 2007;**20**(2):89-100

[59] Arslan E, Yavuz M, Dalay C. The relationship between tumor necrosis factor (TNF)-alpha and survival following granulocyte-colony stimulating factor (G-CSF) administration in burn sepsis. Burns. 2000;**26**(6):521-524

[60] Finnerty CC, Herndon DN, Przkora R, et al. Cytokine expression profile over time in severely burned pediatric patients. Shock. 2006;**26**(1):13-19

[61] Carsin H, Assicot M, Feger F, et al. Evolution and significance of circulating procalcitonin levels compared with IL-6, TNF alpha and endotoxin levels early after thermal injury. Burns. 1997;**23**(3):218-224

[62] Ma L, Zhang H, Yin Y, et al. Role of interleukin-6 to differentiate sepsis from non-infectious systemic inflammatory response syndrome. Cytokine. 2016;**88**:126-135

[63] Kraft R, Herndon DN, Finnerty CC, Cox RA, Song J, Jeschke MG. Predictive value of IL-8 for sepsis and severe infections after burn injury: A clinical study. Shock. 2015;**43**(3):222-227

[64] Csontos C, Foldi V, Palinkas L, et al. Time course of pro- and anti-inflammatory cytokine levels in patients with burns – Prognostic value of interleukin-10. Burns. 2010;**36**(4):483-494

[65] Cakir Madenci O, Yakupoglu S, Benzonana N, Yucel N, Akbaba D, Orcun KA. Evaluation of soluble CD14 subtype (presepsin) in burn sepsis. Burns. 2014;**40**(4):664-669

[66] Zhang J, Hu ZD, Song J, et al. Diagnostic value of Presepsin for sepsis: A systematic review and meta-analysis. Medicine (Baltimore). 2015;**94**:e2158

[67] Barber R, Aragaki C, Rivera-Chavez F, Purdue G, Hunt J, Horton J. TLR4 and TNF-α polymorphisms are associated with an increased risk for severe sepsis following burn injury. Journal of Medical Genetics. 2004;**41**(11):808-813

[68] Bauer M, Giamarellos-Bourboulis EJ, Kortgen A, et al. A transcriptomic biomarker to quantify systemic inflammation in sepsis – A prospective multicentre phase II diagnostic study. eBioMedicine. 2016;**6**:114-125

[69] Mishra J, Mori K, Ma Q, Kelly C, Yang J, Mitsnefes M, et al. Amelioration of ischemic acute renal injury by neutrophil gelatinase-associated lipocalin. J Am Soc Nephrol. Dec 2004;**15**(12):3073-3082

[70] Mishra J, Ma Q, Kelly C, Mitsnefes M, Mori K, Barasch J, et al. Kidney NGAL is a novel early marker of acute injury following transplantation. Pediatric Nephrology. Jun 2006;**21**(6):856-863

[71] Hirsch R, Dent C, Pfriem H, Allen J, Beekman RH 3rd, Ma Q, et al.

NGAL is an early predictive biomarker of contrast-induced nephropathy in children. Pediatric Nephrology. Dec 2007;**22**(12):2089-2095

[72] Han WK, Bailly V, Abichandani R, Thadhani R, Bonventre JV. Kidney injury molecule-1 (KIM-1): A novel biomarker for human renal proximal tubule injury. Kidney International. Jul 2002;**62**(1):237-244

[73] Parikh CR, Jani A, Melnikov VY, Faubel S, Edelstein CL. Urinary interleukin-18 is a marker of human acute tubular necrosis. American Journal of Kidney Diseases. Mar 2004;**43**(3):405-414

[74] Waheed S, Matsushita K, Sang Y, et al. Combined association of albuminuria and cystatin C-based estimated GFR with mortality, coronary heart disease, and heart failure outcomes: the atherosclerosis risk in communities (ARIC) study. American Journal of Kidney Diseases. 2012;**60**:207-216

[75] du Cheyron D, Daubin C, Poggioli J, Ramakers M, Houillier P, Charbonneau P, et al. Urinary measurement of Na+/H+ exchanger isoform 3 (NHE3) protein as new marker of tubule injury in critically ill patients with ARF. American Journal of Kidney Diseases. Sep 2003;**42**(3):497-506

[76] Doi K, Noiri E, Sugaya T. Urinary L-type fatty acid-binding protein as a new renal biomarker in critical care. Current Opinion in Critical Care. 2010 Dec;**16**(6):545-549

[77] Ghajar J. Traumatic brain injury. Lancet. 2000;**356**:923-929

[78] Riggio S, Wong M. Neurobehavioral sequelae of traumatic brain injury. Mt. Sinai J. Med. J. Transl. Pers. Med. 2009;**76**:163-172

[79] Johnson VE, Stewart W, Smith DH. Widespread tau and amyloid-Beta pathology many years after a single traumatic brain injury in humans: Long-term AD-like pathology after single TBI. Brain Pathology. 2012;**22**:142-149

[80] McCrory P, Meeuwisse W, Johnston K, Dvorak J, Aubry M, Molloy M, et al. consensus statement on concussion in sport - the third international conference on concussion in sport held in Zurich, November 2008;Phys. Sportsmed. 2009;**37**:141-159

[81] Sterr A, Herron KA, Hayward C, et al. Are mild head injuries as mild as we think? Neurobehavioral concomitants of chronic post-concussion syndrome. BMC Neurology. 2006;**6**:7 https://doi.org/10.1186/1471-2377-6-7

[82] Bratton SL, Chestnut RM, Ghajar J, McConnell Hammond FF, Harris OA, Hartl R, et al. Guidelines for the management of severe traumatic brain injury. VI. Indications for intracranial pressure monitoring. Journal of Neurotrauma. 2007;**24** (Suppl 1):S37-S44

[83] Kulbe JR, Geddes JW. Current status of fluid biomarkers in mild traumatic brain injury. Experimental Neurology. 2016;**275**:334-352

[84] Calcagnile O, Unden L, Unden J. Clinical validation of S100B use in management of mild head injury. BMC Emergency Medicine. 2012;**12**:13

[85] Bazarian JJ, Merchant-Borna K. Tau, s-100 calcium-binding protein B, and neuron-specific enolase as biomarkers of concussion. JAMA Neurology. 2014 Jul 1;**71**(7):925-926

[86] Bang SA, Song YS, Moon BS, Lee BC, Lee H, Kim J-M, et al. Neuropsychological, metabolic, and GABA A receptor studies in subjects with repetitive traumatic brain injury. Journal of Neurotrauma. 2016;**33**:1005-1014

[87] Zhang Y, Bhavnani BR. Glutamate-induced apoptosis in neuronal cells is mediated via caspase-dependent and independent mechanisms involving calpain and caspase-3 proteases as well as apoptosis inducing factor (AIF) and this process is inhibited by equine oestrogens. BMC Neuroscience. 2006;7:49

[88] Ahmed FA, Kamnaksh A, Kovesdi E, Long JB, Agoston DV. Long-term consequences of single and multiple mild blast exposure on select physiological parameters and blood-based biomarkers. Electrophoresis. 2013;**34**:2229-2233

[89] Walls MK, Race N, Zheng L, Vega-Alvarez SM, Acosta G, Park J, et al. Structural and biochemical abnormalities in the absence of acute deficits in mild primary blast-induced head trauma. Journal of Neurosurgery JNS. 2016;**124**(3):675-686

[90] Harris JL, Yeh H-W, Choi I-Y, Lee P, Berman NE, Swerdlow RH, et al. Altered neurochemical profile after traumatic brain injury: 1H-MRS biomarkers of pathological mechanisms. Journal of Cerebral Blood Flow and Metabolism. 2012;**32**:2122-2134

[91] A Comprehensive Review of the 1H-MRS Metabolite Spectrum in Autism Spectrum Disorder; T.Ford,D. Crewther; Frontiers in Molecular Neuroscience;2016

[92] Plasma neurofilament light as a potential biomarker of neurodegeneration in Alzheimer's disease. Lewczuk P, Ermann N, Andreasson U, Schultheis C, Podhorna J, Spitzer P, Maler JM, Kornhuber J, Blennow K, Zetterberg H. Alzheimer's Research & Therapy 2018 Jul 28; 10(1):71.

[93] Serum neurofilament dynamics predicts neurodegeneration and clinical progression in presymptomatic Alzheimer's disease. Preische O, Schultz SA , Apel A , et al. Nature Medicine 2019;25:277-283.

[94] NIA-AA Research Framework: Toward a biological definition of Alzheimer's disease. Jack CR Jr, Bennett DA, Blennow K, Carrillo MC, Dunn B, Haeberlein SB, Holtzman DM, Jagust W, Jessen F, Karlawish J, Liu E, Molinuevo JL, Montine T, Phelps C, Rankin KP, Rowe CC, Scheltens P, Siemers E, Snyder HM, Sperling R; Alzheimer's & Dementia 2018 Apr; 14(4):535-562.

[95] Phases of A beta-deposition in the human brain and its relevance for the development of AD. Thal DR, Rüb U, Orantes M, Braak H; Neurology 2002 Jun 25; 58(12):1791-1800.

[96] High performance plasma amyloid β biomarkers for Alzheimer's disease. *Nakamura A, Kaneko N, Villemagne VL, Kato T, Doecke J, Doré V, Fowler C, Li QX, Martins R, Rowe C, Tomita T, Matsuzaki K, Ishii K, Ishii K, Arahata Y, Iwamoto S, Ito K, Tanaka K, Masters CL, Yanagisawa K. Nature. 2018 Feb 8; 554(7691):249-254.*

[97] NIA-AA Research Framework: Toward a biological definition of Alzheimer's disease. Jack CR Jr, Bennett DA, Blennow K, Carrillo MC, Dunn B, Haeberlein SB, Holtzman DM, Jagust W, Jessen F, Karlawish J, Liu E, Molinuevo JL, Montine T, Phelps C, Rankin KP, Rowe CC, Scheltens P, Siemers E, Snyder HM, Sperling R. Alzheimer's & Dementia 2018 Apr; 14(4):535-562

[98] Persistent neuropathological effects 14 years following amyloid β immunization in Alzheimer's disease. *Nicoll JAR, Buckland GR, Harrison CH, Page A, Harris S, Love S, Neal JW, Holmes C, Boche D.Brain. 2019 Jul 1; 142(7):2113-2126.*

[99] Association of Plasma Neurofilament Light With Neurodegeneration in Patients With

Alzheimer Disease. *Mattsson N, Andreasson U, Zetterberg H, Blennow K, Alzheimer's Disease Neuroimaging Initiative. JAMA Neurol. 2017 May 1; 74(5):557-566.*

[100] Braak H, Ghebremedhin E, Rub U, Bratzke H, Del Tredici K. Stages in the development of Parkinson's disease-related pathology. Cell and Tissue Research. 2004;**318**(1):121-134. DOI: 10.1007/s00441-004-0956-9

[101] Noyce AJ, Bestwick JP, Silveira-Moriyama L, Hawkes CH, Giovannoni G, Lees AJ, et al. Meta-analysis of early nonmotor features and risk factors for Parkinson disease. Annals of Neurology. 2012;**72**(6):893-901. DOI: 10.1002/ana.23687

[102] Mackenzie IR, Neumann M, Cairns NJ, Munoz DG, Isaacs AM. Novel types of frontotemporal lobar degeneration: Beyond tau and TDP-43. Journal of Molecular Neuroscience. 2011;**45**(3):402-408. DOI: 10.1007/s12031-011-9551-1

[103] Rub U, Seidel K, Heinsen H, Vonsattel JP, den Dunnen WF, Korf HW. Huntington's disease (HD): the neuropathology of a multisystem neurodegenerative disorder of the human brain. Brain Pathology. 2016;**26**(6):726-740. DOI: 10.1111/bpa.12426

[104] A novel pathogenic pathway of immune activation detectable before clinical onset in Huntington's disease. Björkqvist M, Wild EJ, Thiele J, Silvestroni A, Andre R, Lahiri N, Raibon E, Lee RV, Benn CL, Soulet D, Magnusson A, Woodman B, Landles C, Pouladi MA, Hayden MR, Khalili-Shirazi A, Lowdell MW, Brundin P, Bates GP, Leavitt BR, Möller T, Tabrizi SJ; J Exp Med. 2008 Aug 4; 205(8):1869-1877.

[105] The phosphodiesterase 10 positron emission tomography tracer, [18F] MNI-659, as a novel biomarker for early Huntington disease. *Russell DS, Barret O, Jennings DL, Friedman JH, Tamagnan GD, Thomae D, Alagille D, Morley TJ, Papin C, Papapetropoulos S, Waterhouse RN, Seibyl JP, Marek KL. JAMA Neurol. 2014 Dec; 71(12):1520-1528.*

[106] Accuracy of diagnosis criteria in patients with suspected diagnosis of sporadic Creutzfeldt-Jakob disease and detection of 14-3-3 protein, France, 1992 to 2009. *Peckeu L, Delasnerie-Lauprètre N, Brandel JP, Salomon D, Sazdovitch V, Laplanche JL, Duyckaerts C, Seilhean D, Haïk S, Hauw JJ. Euro Surveill. 2017* Oct; *22(41)*

[107] Dynamic changes of oligomeric amyloid β levels in plasma induced by spiked synthetic Aβ42. *An SSA, Lee BS, Yu JS, Lim K, Kim GJ, Lee R, Kim S, Kang S, Park YH, Wang MJ, Yang YS, Youn YC, Kim S; Alzheimers Res Ther. 2017 Oct 17; 9(1):86*

[108] Amyloid β-Secondary Structure Distribution in Cerebrospinal Fluid and Blood Measured by an Immuno-Infrared-Sensor: A biomarker candidate for Alzheimer's Disease.*Nabers A, Ollesch J, Schartner J, Kötting C, Genius J, Hafermann H, Klafki H, Gerwert K, Wiltfang J. Anal Chem. 2016* Mar 1; *88(5):2755-2762*

[109] Locus coeruleus imaging as a biomarker for noradrenergic dysfunction in neurodegenerative diseases. *Betts MJ, Kirilina E, Otaduy MCG, Ivanov D, Acosta-Cabronero J, Callaghan MF et al. Brain. 2019 Sep 1; 142(9):2558-2571*

[110] Schuetz P, Hausfater P, Amin D, et al. Biomarkers from distinct biological pathways improve early risk stratification in medical emergency patients: the multinational, prospective, observational TRIAGE study. Critical Care. 2015;**19**:377

Section 2

Alzheimer's Disease: Molecular Mechanisms, Biomarkers and Treatment

Chapter 4

Alzheimer's Disease and Type 2 Diabetes Mellitus: Molecular Mechanisms and Similarities

Karla Isabel Lira-De León, Alma Delia Bertadillo-Jilote, David Gustavo García-Gutiérrez and Marco Antonio Meraz-Ríos

Abstract

Alzheimer's disease (AD) has become one of the most threatening diseases in the elderly, and type 2 diabetes mellitus (T2DM) is a major health problem in the world, representing 7.4% of the population. Several studies have produced epidemiological, clinical, and pathological evidence of the relationship between AD and T2DM. Laboratory research using animal models has identified mechanisms shared by both T2DM and AD. Particularly, there is an increase of tau phosphorylation and cleavage, which is known to be particularly toxic to neurons and to form a nucleation for neurofibrillary tangles. Also, alterations in synaptic plasticity are associated to tau pathology through the direct abnormal interaction of pathological tau with synaptic proteins and indirectly through Tau-activated neuroinflammatory processes. Many T2DM complications are potentiated or initiated by the accumulation of specific forms of advanced glycation end products (AGEs) and their interaction with its receptors (RAGE). AGEs promote β-amyloid aggregation and cytotoxicity, while glycation of tau may enhance their aggregation. Therefore, this review addresses the analysis of the common mechanisms where the major molecular players of these two diseases participate and contribute to a better understanding of these diseases in their pathogenic relationship.

Keywords: Alzheimer's disease, type 2 diabetes mellitus, metabolic syndrome, β-Amyloid, tau

1. Introduction

Demographic trends show a dramatic increase in the elderly population; unfortunately this group showed a higher prevalence of chronic diseases worldwide, becoming a serious public health problem in both developed and developing countries [1, 2]. The increasing aging population phenomenon in association with chronic diseases has several repercussions: economic, social, and medical. Among these chronic diseases, the most prominent for occupying the first places in epidemiological studies are: cardiovascular, cerebrovascular, diabetes, cancer, and dementias [2, 3].

Diabetes mellitus (DM) is a complex and heterogeneous group characterized by hyperglycemia. In 2015, there were 415 million people with diabetes worldwide and this number is expected to increase to 642 million by 2040 [4, 5]. The major risk factors in DM are eating a diet high in fats and simple sugars coupled with sedentary lifestyle [3]. On the other hand, Alzheimer's disease (AD) is the most common dementia worldwide [6].

Several studies have produced epidemiological, clinical, and pathological evidence of the relationship between AD and DM [7, 8]. It has been reported that patients with diabetes have a 50–75% increased risk of developing AD compared with age- and gender-matched patients without diabetes [9]. In fact, both entities share metabolic dysfunctions associated with different pathological developments [10].

DM is a chronic disease characterized by the absolute or relative shortage of insulin, leading to chronic hyperglycemia, which results either in the progressive failure of pancreatic β-cell function and consequently a lack of insulin production (type 1 diabetes, T1DM) or in the development of insulin resistance and subsequently the loss in β-cell function (type 2 diabetes, T2DM) [4, 11]. Examination of diagnoses reveals that AD is by far the most common cause of dementia among people with T2DM (e.g., 91%) [12]; the insulin resistance in this metabolic disease is not yet clear, but obesity and age are the major risk factors [13, 14].

AD is the most common dementing disorder of late life, characterized by progressive loss of cholinergic neurons and a devastating cognitive decline [10]. The two major histopathological features of AD are: (1) amyloid plaques and (2) neurofibrillary tangles (NFTs). Amyloid plaques are composed of β-amyloid (Aβ) peptide, produced by the proteolytic cleavage of the amyloid precursor protein (APP) [9]. On the other hand, truncated and phosphorylated tau protein is the main component in the NFT and the amount of these aggregates correlates with cognitive impairment [15]. In AD, abnormal tau aggregates are present in the cell body and proximal dendrites [16].

Research studies, using animal models have identified mechanisms that are shared by T2DM and AD [7]. AD pathology has been evaluated extensively in two widely available T2DM spontaneous models: Bio-Breeding Zucker diabetic rat/Wor rats and db/db mice. They observed an increase in tau phosphorylation and cleavage, which is known to be particularly toxic to neurons and forms the nucleation for NFT [9]. The hyperglycemia in T2DM induces an increase in advanced glycation end products (AGEs), and these molecules also accumulate with aging and dementia [17, 18]. AGEs promote Aβ aggregation and cytotoxicity [19], while glycation of tau promotes their aggregation [20].

A fat and simple sugars-rich diet, coupled with sedentary lifestyle, is also a strong risk factor associated with another disorder known as metabolic syndrome (MS), characterized by abdominal obesity, dyslipidemias, high blood pressure, hyperglycemia, insulin resistance, and high body mass index [21–23]. Since many of the characteristic features of MS, including insulin resistance, obesity, dyslipidemia, and high blood pressure, are risk factors not only for DM and cardiovascular disease but also for AD [24], this review will focus on the common mechanisms involved in the development of these diseases.

2. Metabolic syndrome

Metabolic syndrome is a complex disorder defined by a cluster of interconnected factors that increase the risk of cardiovascular atherosclerotic diseases and T2DM [25]. MS is also associated with various cardiometabolic risk factors modulated by several environmental conditions, mainly an inadequate diet and physical inactivity [26]. The syndrome presents simultaneously with insulin resistance, alterations in blood glucose levels, hypertension, triglycerides above normal, levels below recommended of high density lipoprotein (cHDL), and visceral obesity [22]. The process starts with an inadequate diet as well as a sedentary life, which induce the development of obesity, usually with episodes of hyperinsulinemia, which in turn can produce insulin resistance due to the blockade of insulin receptors and glucose transporters, with the presence of high levels of fatty acids and glucose in the extracellular space (associated with DM), associated with hypertension and low synthesis and increased triglyceride catabolism. There are also dyslipidemias due to the inability to inhibit lipolysis in fatty tissues, with an increase in low-density lipoprotein (cLDL) and a decrease in cHDL. Finally, obesity develops due to the continuous increase in visceral fat, a permanent pro-inflammatory state, and endothelial dysfunction [27].

2.1 Etiology

The etiology of MS is attributed to the combination of genetic and environmental factors associated with lifestyles.

Obesity is "a chronic, relapsing, multifactorial, neurobehavioral disease, wherein an increase in body fat promotes adipose tissue dysfunction and abnormal fat mass physical forces, resulting in adverse metabolic, biomechanical, and psychosocial health consequences." Includes the increase and accumulation of fat at the visceral level (fatty tissue deposit mainly in the liver, intestine and pancreas), the tissue is rich in macrophages; adipocytes produce a variety of biologically active molecules, known together as adipokines [28].

Dyslipidemia is a disorder of lipoprotein metabolism, including lipoprotein overproduction or deficiency. Dyslipidemias may be manifested by elevation of the total cholesterol, the "bad" cLDL cholesterol and the triglyceride concentrations, and a decrease in the "good" cHDL cholesterol concentration in the blood. Dyslipidemia has been attributed to the inability of insulin to inhibit lipolysis at the level of adipose tissue, which leads to an increase in the release of free fatty acids and a greater contribution of these to the liver, inducing increased apolipoprotein B secretion [29].

Hypertension, also known as high or raised blood pressure, is a condition in which the blood vessels have persistently raised pressure. Hypertension is produced as a consequence of the effects of the hyperinsulinemia. The blood pressure rises, due to an increase in the reabsorption of sodium and water in the renal proximal tubule. Hyperinsulinemia also increases peripheral vascular resistance and increases the activation of the sympathetic system with the consequent increase in circulating catecholamines and stimulation of the renin angiotensin-aldosterone system [30].

Hyperglycemia is the technical term for high blood glucose blood sugar. High blood sugar happens when the body has too little insulin or when the body cannot use insulin properly. This poor insulin secretion or action is due to lipotoxicity of the pancreatic β cells, since the excessive accumulation of triglycerides in pancreatic islets increases the expression of the inducible nitric oxide synthase (iNOS) enzyme, increasing nitric oxide levels and producing impaired function and finally apoptosis. The β cells, progressively losing its ability to compensate the insulin resistance with more insulin secretion, and finally increasing blood glucose levels [31].

Insulin resistance is defined clinically as the inability of a known quantity of exogenous or endogenous insulin to increase glucose uptake and utilization in an individual as much as it does in a normal population. Insulin action is the consequence of insulin binding to its plasma membrane receptor and the signal is transmitted through the cell by a series of protein–protein interactions. Classically, this refers to impaired sensitivity to insulin-mediated glucose disposal. Compensatory hyperinsulinemia occurs when pancreatic β cell secretion increases to maintain normal blood glucose levels in the setting of peripheral insulin resistance in muscle and adipose tissue [32].

Pro-inflammatory states acute and chronic hyperglycemias are pro-inflammatory states, central obesity and insulin resistance being implicated in its etiology. Adipose tissue is biologically active as an endocrine and paracrine organ. Adipocytes undergo hypertrophy and hyperplasia in response to nutritional excess that can lead the cells to outgrow their blood supply with induction of a hypoxic state. Hypoxia can lead to cell necrosis with macrophage infiltration and the production of adipokines, which include the pro-inflammatory mediators interleukin-6 (IL-6) and tumor necrosis factor alpha (TNF-α), as well as the prothrombotic mediator plasminogen activator inhibitor-1 (PAI-1, [33]). These mediators induce an oxidative stress and endothelial dysfunction, and nitric oxide (NO) regulates the vascular tone by activating guanylate cyclase and increasing the 3′5′-guanosine monophosphate and inhibits platelet activity. When there is an excessive production of superoxide anion, the bioavailability of NO decreases due to their oxidative inactivation in the vascular wall [34].

2.2 Diagnosis of metabolic syndrome

The diagnostic criteria of the MS have been subject to many definitions, such as those of World Health Organization (WHO), Adult Treatment Panel III of the National Cholesterol Education Program (ATP III), International Diabetes Federation (IDF), American Heart Association (AHA) and others. However, a new global definition of the metabolic syndrome was proposed by the IDF where obesity represents a necessary requirement for the diagnosis of MS. Once the obesity is confirmed, the diagnosis continues with the presence of two or more parameters such as decrease in cHDL and increase in triglyceride, blood pressure and blood glucose [35–37]. However, even with a good diagnosis for MS, in most cases the treatment is inadequate [38].

Several MS components are present in AD and T2DM, including insulin resistance, obesity, dyslipidemia, and high blood pressure [24]. These common mechanisms are required to be analyzed deeper, and how each one of them contributes in all these pathologies should be described.

3. Amyloid forming diseases

AD and T2DM are amyloid forming diseases characterized by the presence of insoluble protein aggregates with a fibrillary conformation in brain and pancreas, respectively [39].

The presence of proteinaceous plaques that primarily comprise islet amyloid polypeptide (IAPP, one of the major secretory products of the pancreatic β-cells) is found in the majority of patients (approximately 90%) with T2DM [40]. Although it is not clear why normally soluble IAPP can form toxic aggregates, the evidence suggests that the presence of an amyloidogenic sequence in the IAPP molecule could increase the IAPP production/secretion from β-cells associated with elevated insulin demand and abnormalities in trafficking/processing of pro-IAPP contribute to aggregation in T2DM, causing cellular dysfunction and consequent membrane disruption, channel formation and toxicity [41]. Further, several groups have found that Aβ1–42 and IAPP forms form early intermediate assemblies as spherical oligomers, implicating a common folding pattern (**Figure 1**, [42]).

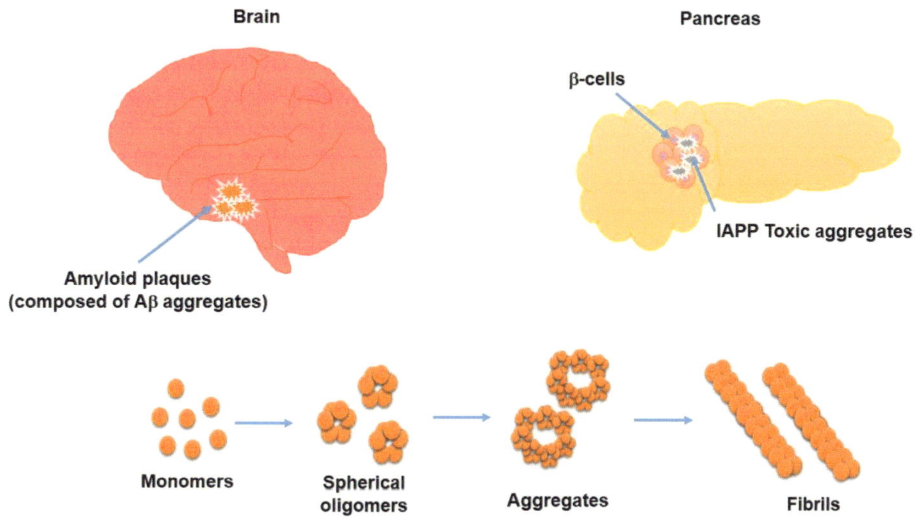

Figure 1.
Common ways of amyloid toxicity in Alzheimer's disease and type 2 diabetes mellitus. Insoluble protein aggregates with a fibrillary conformation are present in both entities, causing cell death in neurons and β-cells of brain and pancreas, respectively.

4. Insulin alterations

In addition to T2DM (insulin resistance), T1DM (insulin deficiency) shares mechanisms with AD, and researchers have called the set of these characteristics type 3 diabetes. Defects in insulin signaling causes alterations in glucose metabolism and leads to an energy imbalance causing the production of reactive oxygen species (ROS), DNA damage, and mitochondrial dysfunction; all these cascades lead to pro-apoptosis, pro-inflammatory and production of toxic peptides (tau and Aβ) [43].

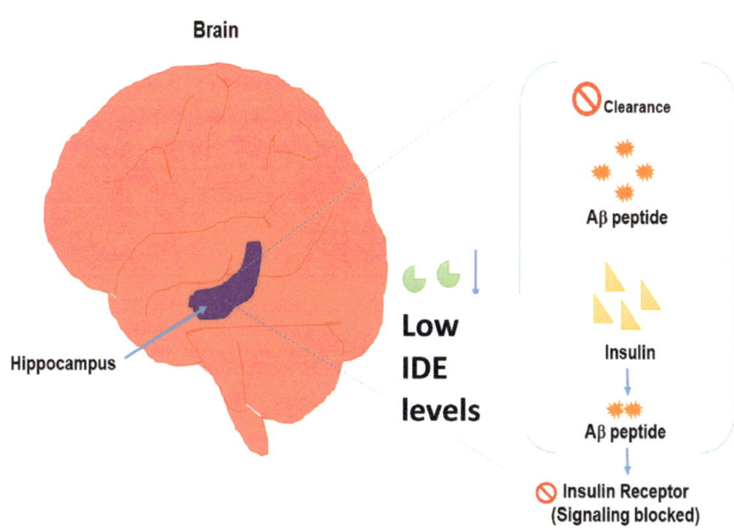

Figure 2.
Abnormal clearance of toxic species of β-amyloid by insulin degrading enzyme. Hippocampus with decreased levels of insulin degrading enzyme (IDE) leads to Aβ accumulation, which blocks the insulin receptor signaling, altering synaptic plasticity and architecture of dendritic spines.

Insulin regulates glucose metabolism in peripheral tissues and also affects brain functions including cognition, memory, and synaptic plasticity through complex insulin/insulin receptor (IR) signaling pathways [44]. Insulin resistance in the brain is presented by reduced levels of insulin and insulin growth factor (IGF) receptors. Insulin and IGF deficiency are associated with an altered expression of insulin and IGF polypeptides in the brain and cerebrospinal fluid (CSF), which causes accumulation of Aβ [45]. On the other hand, chronic peripheral hyperinsulinemia and central insulin resistance can modulate tau phosphorylation, and with the loss of insulin-like growth factor 1 (IGF-1) signaling, an increase in tau hyperphosphorylation and NFT formation has been observed [46]. Through the inhibition of insulin signaling, Akt kinase is also inhibited, which in turn activates the glycogen synthase kinase 3β (GSK3ß), probably causing an increase of tau phosphorylation and altering its binding to microtubules [9].

Insulin degrading enzyme (IDE) is a major factor responsible for insulin degradation. However, IDE degrades other targets like glucagon, atrial natriuretic peptide, and Aβ, and this could be another connection between T2DM and AD. The decrease of IDE in the hippocampus has been associated with a greater susceptibility of this region to the accumulation of Aβ (**Figure 2**, [47]).

5. Hyperglycemia

The T2DM patients have chronic hyperglycemia with an impaired glucose metabolism (poor glucose transport), altering neuronal cell and their metabolism contribute to AD. In patients with AD, a decrease in glucose metabolism has been observed, typically identified with fluorodeoxyglucose positron emission tomography (PET), even before clinical symptoms of dementia were present [48].

Deficits in glucose metabolism might also potentiate the neuronal cell death produced by other pathological processes (such as abnormal cholesterol metabolism or high levels of Aβ), which in turn might be influenced by genetic predisposition such as possession of Apolipoprotein E ε4 (APOE ε4) alleles [49].

It is generally accepted that many DM complications are potentiated or initiated by the accumulation of specific forms of AGEs and their interaction with its receptors (RAGE). The AGEs are molecules (including peptides and proteins) formed as a result of the Maillard reaction. In T2DM, periods of hyperglycemia induce an increase in AGEs formation, although these molecules also accumulate with aging accelerated formation [17, 18]. AGEs promote Aβ aggregation and cytotoxicity [19] and glycation of tau may enhance their aggregation as well [20].

6. Dyslipidemia

Cholesterol may be directly involved in Aβ aggregation, by abnormal oxidative metabolites such as cholesterol-derived aldehydes, which can promote the amyloidogenesis process. Also, it was observed that APOE ε4, cholesterol, and Aβ are components of the amyloid plaques both in humans and animal models of AD. Further, low levels of cholesterol affect APP metabolism, with an increase in the secretion of soluble APP, a non-amyloidogenic soluble N-terminal derivative, also found in human CSF [50].

7. Obesity

The mechanism for the association between obesity and dementia is still far from being understood. Whitmer et al. alluded to the involvement of adiposity with inflammation and its markers [51] while Liu et al. report that obesity also has been related with defective brain insulin signaling in experimental models and postmortem brains [52]. This is important because there have been several reports where insulin regulates synaptic plasticity through altering internalization of neurotransmitter receptors, in the cortex and hippocampus, which are regions of the brain generally associated with learning and memory, respectively [14, 53]. Therefore, alterations in synaptic plasticity may be associated to tau pathology, through a direct abnormal interaction of pathological tau species with synaptic proteins but also indirectly through tau-activated neuroinflammatory processes [54].

Another possible mechanism linking obesity with dementia is the oxidative stress, resulting from an increased intake of sugars and fats, which is the hallmark of the modern diet [55, 56]. Rats maintained on a diet high in refined sugar and rich in fat generated higher concentrations of free radicals [51]. Inflammatory processes promote vascular complications in obesity, T2DM, and AD. The primary regulator of this response is NF-κB, and in these pathologies there is an increase of the NF-κB family of transcription factors. In AD, the reactive astrocytes in close proximity to the Aβ plaques produce inflammatory cytokines, including IL-1β and TNF-α, and inducible iNOS, which generate free radicals such as NO, that can be neurotoxic [38].

8. Hypertension

Mice that have been chronically subjected to high blood pressure show deposition of amyloid aggregates and loss of memory when they are examined in specific tasks. Besides this, the hypertensive challenge increases the expression of RAGE, leading to Aβ deposition and learning impairment [57, 58].

A few autopsy studies have showed that the severity of AD pathology is increased by the presence of cerebrovascular damage, which is strongly linked to hypertension [58, 59].

Chronic hypertension induced vascular abnormalities in the brain, such as increased vascular stiffness, and decreased vessel wall plasticity; this alters arterial pulsations, disturbing the glymphatic system and leading to a significant increase of Aβ deposition in the brain parenchyma [60]. The glymphatic system is a macroscopic waste clearance system that utilizes a unique system of perivascular tunnels, formed by astroglial cells, to promote efficient elimination of soluble proteins and metabolites from the central nervous system [61].

Cerebral amyloid angiopathy has been shown to interact with amyloid plaques and NFT and to increase the severity of cognitive impairment beyond that seen in people with each histopathological feature separately [62].

9. Conclusion

There are several mechanisms in common between AD and T2DM, and a better understanding of their interrelation would contribute to upgrade the control of these diseases. Working in this direction will be important in order to identify new therapeutic or common targets, especially before the most severe symptoms of both pathologies occur. In addition to better management of the patients, this will improve the patient's quality of life.

Conflict of interest

The authors declare no conflict of interest.

Author details

Karla Isabel Lira-De León[1], Alma Delia Bertadillo-Jilote[1], David Gustavo García-Gutiérrez[1] and Marco Antonio Meraz-Ríos[2]*

1 Faculty of Chemistry, Autonomous University of Queretaro, Queretaro, Mexico

2 Department of Molecular Biomedicine, Center for Research and Advanced Studies of the National Polytechnic Institute (CINVESTAV-IPN), Mexico City, Mexico

*Address all correspondence to: mmeraz@cinvestav.mx

References

[1] Chapel JM, Ritchey MD, Zhang D, et al. Prevalence and medical costs of chronic diseases among adult Medicaid beneficiaries. American Journal of Preventive Medicine. 2017;**53**:S143-S154

[2] Maresova P, Javanmardi E, Barakovic S, et al. Consequences of chronic diseases and other limitations associated with old age—A scoping review. BMC Public Health. 2019;**19**:1431

[3] Mastrangelo A, Barbas C. Chronic diseases and lifestyle biomarkers identification by metabolomics. Advances in Experimental Medicine and Biology. 2017;**965**:235-263

[4] Rawshani A, Rawshani A, Franzén S, et al. Mortality and cardiovascular disease in type 1 and type 2 diabetes. The New England Journal of Medicine. 2017;**376**:1407-1418

[5] Koye DN, Magliano DJ, Nelson RG, et al. The global epidemiology of diabetes and kidney disease. Advances in Chronic Kidney Disease. 2018;**25**:121-132

[6] Robinson M, Lee BY, Hane FT. Recent Progress in Alzheimer's disease research, part 2: Genetics and epidemiology. Journal of Alzheimer's Disease. 2017;**57**:317-330

[7] Park SA. A common pathogenic mechanism linking type-2 diabetes and Alzheimer's disease: Evidence from animal models. Journal of Clinical Neurology. 2011;7:10-18

[8] Correia SC, Santos RX, Carvalho C, et al. Insulin signaling, glucose metabolism and mitochondria: Major players in Alzheimer's disease and diabetes interrelation. Brain Research. 2012;**1441**:64-78

[9] Kim B, Backus C, Oh S, et al. Increased tau phosphorylation and cleavage in mouse models of type 1 and type 2 diabetes. Endocrinology. 2009;**150**:5294-5301

[10] Domínguez RO, Marschoff ER, González SE, et al. Type 2 diabetes and/or its treatment leads to less cognitive impairment in Alzheimer's disease patients. Diabetes Research and Clinical Practice. 2012;**98**:68-74

[11] Lu J, Xie G, Jia W, et al. Metabolomics in human type 2 diabetes research. Frontiers in Medicine. 2013;**7**:4-13

[12] Luchsinger JA, Tang M-X, Shea S, et al. Hyperinsulinemia and risk of Alzheimer disease. Neurology. 2004;**63**:1187-1192

[13] Naseer MI, Bibi F, Alqahtani MH, et al. Role of gut microbiota in obesity, type 2 diabetes and Alzheimer's disease. CNS & Neurological Disorders Drug Targets. 2014;**13**:305-311

[14] Chen Y, Yu Q, Gong C-X. Molecular connection between diabetes and dementia. Advances in Experimental Medicine and Biology. 2019;**1128**:103-131

[15] Gendron TF, Petrucelli L. The role of tau in neurodegeneration. Molecular Neurodegeneration. 2009;**4**:13

[16] Šimić G, Babić Leko M, Wray S, et al. Tau protein hyperphosphorylation and aggregation in Alzheimer's disease and other tauopathies, and possible neuroprotective strategies. Biomolecules. 2016;**6**. DOI: 10.3390/biom6010006. Epub ahead of print 6 January 2016

[17] Bucala R, Cerami A. Advanced glycosylation: Chemistry, biology, and implications for diabetes and aging. Advances in Pharmacology. 1992;**23**:1-34

[18] Sato T, Shimogaito N, Wu X, et al. Toxic advanced glycation end products (TAGE) theory in Alzheimer's disease. American Journal of Alzheimer's Disease and Other Dementias. 2006;**21**:197-208

[19] Woltjer RL, Maezawa I, Ou JJ, et al. Advanced glycation endproduct precursor alters intracellular amyloid-beta/a beta PP carboxy-terminal fragment aggregation and cytotoxicity. Journal of Alzheimer's Disease. 2003;**5**:467-476

[20] Kuhla B, Haase C, Flach K, et al. Effect of pseudophosphorylation and cross-linking by lipid peroxidation and advanced glycation end product precursors on tau aggregation and filament formation. The Journal of Biological Chemistry. 2007;**282**:6984-6991

[21] Patterson R, McNamara E, Tainio M, et al. Sedentary behaviour and risk of all-cause, cardiovascular and cancer mortality, and incident type 2 diabetes: A systematic review and dose response meta-analysis. European Journal of Epidemiology. 2018;**33**:811-829

[22] Li Y, Zhao L, Yu D, et al. Metabolic syndrome prevalence and its risk factors among adults in China: A nationally representative cross-sectional study. PLOS One. 2018;**13**. DOI: 10.1371/journal.pone.0199293. Epub ahead of print 19 June 2018

[23] Jeong H-S. The relationship between workplace environment and metabolic syndrome. International Journal of Occupational and Environmental Medicine. 2018;**9**:176-183

[24] Martins IJ, Hone E, Foster JK, et al. Apolipoprotein E, cholesterol metabolism, diabetes, and the convergence of risk factors for Alzheimer's disease and cardiovascular disease. Molecular Psychiatry. 2006;**11**:721-736

[25] Kassi E, Pervanidou P, Kaltsas G, et al. Metabolic syndrome: Definitions and controversies. BMC Medicine. 2011;**9**:48

[26] Pacheco-Armenta MC, Jáquez-Torres JÁ. Prevalencia de síndrome metabólico en la consulta externa. Revista de Sanidad Militar. 2017;**71**:264-275

[27] Laclaustra Gimeno M, Bergua Martínez C, Pascual Calleja I, et al. Síndrome metabólico. Concepto y fisiopatología. Revista Española de Cardiología. 2005;**5**:3D-10D

[28] Després J-P, Lemieux I. Abdominal obesity and metabolic syndrome. Nature. 2006;**444**:881-887

[29] Chen D, Zhao X, Sui Z, et al. A multi-omics investigation of the molecular characteristics and classification of six metabolic syndrome relevant diseases. Theranostics. 2020;**10**:2029-2046

[30] Kulkarni H, Mamtani M, Blangero J, et al. Lipidomics in the study of hypertension in metabolic syndrome. Current Hypertension Reports. 2017;**19**:7

[31] Shah SS, Ramirez CE, Powers AC, et al. Hyperglycemic clamp-derived disposition index is negatively associated with metabolic syndrome severity in obese subjects. Metabolism, Clinical and Experimental. 2016;**65**:835-842

[32] Wilcox G. Insulin and insulin resistance. Clinical Biochemist Reviews. 2005;**26**:19-39

[33] McCracken E, Monaghan M, Sreenivasan S. Pathophysiology of the metabolic syndrome. Clinics in Dermatology. 2018;**36**:14-20

[34] Carrier A. Metabolic syndrome and oxidative stress: A complex relationship.

Antioxidants & Redox Signaling. 2017;**26**:429-431

[35] Sherling DH, Perumareddi P, Hennekens CH. Metabolic syndrome. Journal of Cardiovascular Pharmacology and Therapeutics. 2017;**22**:365-367

[36] Rochlani Y, Pothineni NV, Kovelamudi S, et al. Metabolic syndrome: Pathophysiology, management, and modulation by natural compounds. Therapeutic Advances in Cardiovascular Disease. 2017;**11**:215-225

[37] Zimmet P, MM Alberti KG, Serrano Ríos M. Una nueva definición mundial del síndrome metabólico propuesta por la Federación Internacional de Diabetes: Fundamento y resultados. Revista Española de Cardiología. 2005;**58**:1371-1376

[38] Friedrich N. Metabolomics in diabetes research. The Journal of Endocrinology. 2012;**215**:29-42

[39] Ashraf GM, Greig NH, Khan TA, et al. Protein misfolding and aggregation in Alzheimer's disease and type 2 diabetes mellitus. CNS & Neurological Disorders Drug Targets. 2014;**13**:1280-1293

[40] Höppener JW, Ahrén B, Lips CJ. Islet amyloid and type 2 diabetes mellitus. The New England Journal of Medicine. 2000;**343**:411-419

[41] Wu C, Shea J-E. Structural similarities and differences between amyloidogenic and non-amyloidogenic islet amyloid polypeptide (IAPP) sequences and implications for the dual physiological and pathological activities of these peptides. PLoS Computational Biology. 2013;**9**:e1003211

[42] Green JD, Goldsbury C, Kistler J, et al. Human amylin oligomer growth and fibril elongation define two distinct phases in amyloid formation. The Journal of Biological Chemistry. 2004;**279**:12206-12212

[43] Calvo-Ochoa E, Heras-Sandoval D, Arias C. Diabetes tipo 3: Resistencia a insulina y enfermedad de Alzheimer. Archivos de Neurociencias. 2016;**21**:83

[44] Calsolaro V, Edison P. Alterations in glucose metabolism in Alzheimer's disease. Recent Patents on Endocrine, Metabolic & Immune Drug Discovery. 2016;**10**:31-39

[45] Jagua Gualdrón A, Ávila Ávila V. Insulin and Alzheimer disease: Type 3 diabetes? Revista de la Facultad de Medicina. 2007;**55**:66-70

[46] Cheng C, Tseng V, Wang J, et al. Tau is hyperphosphorylated in the insulin-like growth factor-I null brain. Endocrinology. 2006;**146**:5086-5091

[47] Pivovarova O, Höhn A, Grune T, et al. Insulin-degrading enzyme: New therapeutic target for diabetes and Alzheimer's disease? Annals of Medicine. 2016;**48**:614-624

[48] Wang T, Huang Q, Reiman EM, et al. Effects of memantine on clinical ratings, fluorodeoxyglucose positron emission tomography measurements, and cerebrospinal fluid assays in patients with moderate to severe Alzheimer dementia: A 24-week, randomized, clinical trial. Journal of Clinical Psychopharmacology. 2013;**33**:636-642

[49] Liao F, Yoon H, Kim J. Apolipoprotein E metabolism and functions in brain and its role in Alzheimer's disease. Current Opinion in Lipidology. 2017;**28**:60-67

[50] Wang C, Shou Y, Pan J, et al. The relationship between cholesterol level and Alzheimer's disease-associated APP proteolysis/Aβ metabolism. Nutritional Neuroscience. 2019;**22**:453-463

[51] Tabet N. Obesity in middle age and future risk of dementia: Dietary fat and sugar may hold the clue. BMJ. 2005;**331**:454-455; author reply 455

[52] Liu Y, Liu F, Grundke-Iqbal I, et al. Deficient brain insulin signalling pathway in Alzheimer's disease and diabetes. The Journal of Pathology. 2011;**225**:54-62

[53] Cole AR, Astell A, Green C, et al. Molecular connexions between dementia and diabetes. Neuroscience and Biobehavioral Reviews. 2007;**31**:1046-1063

[54] Blum D, Buée L. Alzheimer's disease risk, obesity and tau: Is insulin resistance guilty? Expert Review of Neurotherapeutics. 2013;**13**:461-463

[55] Perez-Martinez P, Phillips CM, Delgado-Lista J, et al. Nutrigenetics, metabolic syndrome risk and personalized nutrition. Current Vascular Pharmacology. 2013;**11**:946-953

[56] Razay G, Raza G, Vreugdenhil A. Obesity in middle age and future risk of dementia: Midlife obesity increases risk of future dementia. BMJ. 2005;**331**:455; author reply 455

[57] Carnevale D, Perrotta M, Lembo G, et al. Pathophysiological links among hypertension and Alzheimer's disease. High Blood Pressure & Cardiovascular Prevention. 2016;**23**:3-7

[58] Marfany A, Sierra C, Camafort M, et al. High blood pressure, Alzheimer disease and antihypertensive treatment. Panminerva Medica. 2018;**60**:8-16

[59] Morris MC, Scherr PA, Hebert LE, et al. Association of incident Alzheimer disease and blood pressure measured from 13 years before to 2 years after diagnosis in a large community study. Archives of Neurology. 2001;**58**:1640-1646

[60] Niwa K, Kazama K, Younkin L, et al. Cerebrovascular autoregulation is profoundly impaired in mice overexpressing amyloid precursor protein. American Journal of Physiology. Heart and Circulatory Physiology. 2002;**283**:H315-H323

[61] Jessen NA, Munk ASF, Lundgaard I, et al. The glymphatic system: A beginner's guide. Neurochemical Research. 2015;**40**:2583-2599

[62] Vagelatos NT, Eslick GD. Type 2 diabetes as a risk factor for Alzheimer's disease: The confounders, interactions, and neuropathology associated with this relationship. Epidemiologic Reviews. 2013;**35**:152-160

Chapter 5

EEG Biomarker for Alzheimer's Disease

Demet Ilhan Algin, Demet Ozbabalık Adapinar and Oguz Osman Erdinc

Abstract

Alzheimer's disease (AD) is a neurodegenerative disorder that accounts for nearly 70% of the more than 50 million dementia cases estimated worldwide. There is no cure for AD. Currently, AD diagnosis is carried out using neuropsychological tests, neuroimaging scans, and laboratory tests. In the early stages of AD, brain computed tomography (CT) and magnetic resonance imaging (MRI) findings may be normal, but in late periods, diffuse cortical atrophy can be detected more prominently in the temporal and frontal regions. Electroencephalogram (EEG) is a test that records the electrical signals of the brain by using electrodes that directly reflects cortical neuronal functioning. In addition, EEG is noninvasive and widely available at low cost, has high resolution, and provides access to neuronal signals, unlike functional MR or PET which indirectly detects metabolic signals. Accurate, specific, and cost-effective biomarkers are needed to track the early diagnosis, progression, and treatment response of AD. The findings of EEG in AD are now identified as biomarkers. In this chapter, we reviewed studies that used EEG or event-related potential (ERP) indices as a biomarker of AD.

Keywords: Alzheimer's disease, biomarker, EEG, quantitative EEG, neurodegeneration

1. Introduction

Alzheimer's disease (AD) is a neurodegenerative disease that accounts for about 70% of the estimated 46 million dementia cases worldwide. Although there is no definitive treatment for AD, early diagnosis and correct follow-up to stop disease progression can improve the quality of life for the AD patients and caregivers [1].

Amnesia, aphasia, apraxia, and agnosia are the leading clinical signs of AD. The first symptom in AD is often the loss of the ability to learn new information (amnesia). Loss of episodic memory is the main symptom of AD. Episodic memory is particularly concerned with the hippocampus. In the beginning, the patient becomes forgetful, repeats the same things, and loses his things. Semantic memory is about social events and general knowledge. It is not destroyed as markedly as episodic memory in the early stages of AD. As the disease progresses, destruction starts in semantic memory [2–4].

According to the symptomatology, AD is divided into three stages: (1) preclinical, (2) mild cognitive impairment (MCI), and (3) AD-related dementia. (1) Preclinical AD: changes in brain, blood, and cerebrospinal fluid associated with AD begin to occur, but the patient does not show any symptoms. This stage may start years or decades before the first clinical symptoms of dementia [5]. (2) Mild cognitive impairment (MCI): MCI describes the clinical situation between normal aging and Alzheimer's disease. In 1999, the information that memory impairment differs according to age, as well as educational level, was added to the definition made on MCI. MCI usually manifests itself with subjective complaints such as forgetting the names and not being able to remember where the items were placed. However, it has been observed that 30% of cases diagnosed with MCI do not progress to AD soon [6]. (3) Alzheimer's dementia: Typically, the symptoms of the disease begin with mild memory difficulties and cognitive impairment develops into dysfunctions in complex daily activities and some other aspects of cognition. When AD is diagnosed clinically, neuron loss and neuropathological lesions occur in many brain regions [7]. However, there is no ideal biomarker to identify AD, and a definitive diagnosis can only be made by autopsy or biopsy. Therefore, the diagnosis of AD can be made by medical history, laboratory tests, neuroimaging, and neuropsychological methods. These clinical assessments are not specific and costly. As a result, an accurate, universal, specific, and cost-effective biomarker is needed for early diagnosis and to monitor disease progression and treatment response [8].

The National Institute on Aging-Alzheimer's Association (NIA-AA) has developed new study criteria to use a panel of prognostic fluids and imaging biomarkers to determine the probability of AD pathology and preclinical AD staging and prodromal and later progression to clinical AD. These are cerebrospinal fluid (CSF) amyloid-β (Aβ) 42, amyloid positron emission tomography (PET), CSF total tau, threonine 181 (T181) phospho-tau, magnetic resonance imaging (MRI) mesial temporal lobe (MTL) atrophy, 18F-fluorodeoxyglucose (FDG)-PET temporoparietal/precuneus hypometabolism, or hypoperfusion [9]. Today, standard neuropsychological tests are used to diagnose AD and are widely supported by expensive neuroimaging methods and invasive laboratory tests. In recent years, electroencephalography (EEG) has emerged as an alternative noninvasive technique compared to more expensive neuroimaging methods such as MRI and PET [10, 11].

2. Alzheimer's disease and its pathophysiology

Data obtained with AD have shown the presence of amyloid plaques and neurofibrillary tangles in the pathology of the disease and that these pathological aggregates have a specific distribution pattern and density [12, 13].

Molecular studies have shown that the main component of amyloid plaques is amyloid beta (Aβ), and neurofibrillary tangles are tau protein. In AD patients, the pathway that forms the Aβ peptide is more active or is thought to be a defect in the mechanism of Aβ clearance. There are mature fibrils in the structure of amyloid plaques. In pathology studies in AD patients, amyloid plaques are indispensable pathological findings and Aβ formation in the pathogenesis of the disease is thought to initiate the pathogenesis of the disease. This hypothesis is defined as the "amyloid cascade hypothesis" [14]. In the pathogenesis of AD, tau hyperphosphorylation is known to impair microtubule stability and function, as well as to gain toxic function, for instance, tau aggregates induce apoptosis. However, like Aβ, it is thought that the tau oligomers they form are associated with neurodegeneration and memory impairment rather than the aggregates formed by the tau protein [15].

3. Alzheimer's disease and EEG

The source of routine EEG activity recorded from the scalp is the postsynaptic potentials of cortical pyramidal cells. According to the synaptic activity being excitatory and inhibitory, the postsynaptic membrane becomes depolarized or hyperpolarized. The total electrical current generated by these excitatory and inhibitory postsynaptic potentials from millions of neurons creates superficial EEG activity. Adeli and Ghosh-Dastidar developed the wavelet-chaos method for the analysis of delta, theta, alpha, and beta (**Table 1**) subbands of EEG to identify potential markers in Alzheimer's disease.

To evaluate the effect of visual warning and attention, evaluation is done with eyes open and eyes closed. EEGs from different loci in the brain are used to explore the responsible areas of the brain and directly measure the functioning of synapses in real time [16, 17].

In AD, a significant decrease in cortical alpha frequency (8–10.5 Hz) was observed, especially in the limbic, temporal, parietal, and central areas [6]. However, it has been reported that the age of onset of AD can change this criterion, and that focal and diffuse EEG abnormalities are more common in early onset AD patients than in late-age AD patients. In the first studies, an increase in theta activity in EEG was considered as one of the earliest changes in Alzheimer's dementia, while alpha activity was found to decrease during or after the disease [18].

EEG markers showing the progression of the disease in MCI cases include an increase in delta and theta power and a decrease in beta or alpha power in the temporal and occipital regions [19]. Osipova et al. showed that alpha rhythm shifts from the parieto-occipital region to temporal regions in AD [20]. In other spontaneous EEG studies, it was found that frontal delta and occipital theta sources were higher in MCI patients than healthy ones, and frontal delta sources and the Mini-Mental State Examination (MMSE) showed negative correlations [21, 22].

The cortical cholinergic system has an important role in controlling many different functions such as cerebral blood flow, cortical activity, sleep/wake cycle, modulation of cortical plasticity, and cognitive performance and learning-memory processes. The presence of cholinergic neurons in the basal forebrain was first reported by Shute and Lewis in 1967. ACh deficiency is observed in the brains of individuals with AD in the entire cortex, especially the temporoparietal cortex [23, 24]. Also, one of the possible mechanisms underlying the observed relationship between Aβ42 and increased slow EEG activity is Aβ and cholinergic deficiencies in the brain in AD. Cholinergic therapy has different effects on delta and theta oscillation responses. Theta oscillations were similar in controls to those receiving cholinergic therapy in the AD patients, regardless of treatment. In other words, theta oscillation responses are affected by cholinergic therapy in AD patients, while the amplitudes of delta oscillation responses are not affected by cholinergic therapy [25].

Moreover, in studies evaluating the relationship between AD neuropathology, EEG frequencies, and CSF markers, amyloid β42 (Aβ42) showed a significant relationship with slow frequency (delta and theta) activity, while phospho-tau (p-tau) and total tau (t-tau) are associated with activity at only fast frequencies (alpha and beta) (26). Smailovic et al. demonstrated the correlation of qEEG and

Type of wave	Frequency
Beta	>13 Hz
Alpha	8–13 Hz
Theta	4–7 Hz
Delta	1–4 Hz

Table 1.
EEG waves.

CSF abnormalities with the AD profile at different stages of cognitive impairment, which revealed that qEEG can demonstrate neurodegeneration-induced synaptic dysfunction [26].

4. Sensory-stimulated oscillations

Sensory-evoked oscillatory responses are obtained by digital filtering of the frequency bands such as delta, theta, alpha, beta, and gamma of the "evoked potential" that appears with the delivery of the sensory stimulus. Haupt et al. showed that gamma and beta2 bands showed a different distribution compared to both patient groups in the visual-evoked oscillatory responses that they examined in Alzheimer's, MCI and healthy group controls, and the current density distribution followed a movement from the right hemisphere to the left hemisphere in these patient groups. In a visual sensory-evoked oscillatory study, the difference between AD patients and the healthy group was shown to disappear when the stimulus did not contain the cognitive load. Besides, when controlled, the parieto-occipital theta-stimulated oscillatory responses of the untreated Alzheimer's patient group were found to be higher than those of the treated Alzheimer's patient group and the healthy group [27].

5. Sensory-evoked coherencies and event-related coherences

Coherence or phase-locking statistics are the most common methods used to evaluate relationships between neural communities [28, 29]. Hogan et al. investigated memory-related EEG strength and coherence in the temporal and central areas in early stage AD patients and the normal control group and the behavioral performances of mild Alzheimer patients did not differ significantly from the healthy ones while they found a decrease in high alpha coherence between central and right temporal cortex of Alzheimer patients [30]. Rossini et al. measured the spontaneous EEG coherence of healthy control and MCI patients (progressive and constant) and found that the course of disease in patients with high coherence in the delta and gamma frequency bands progressed faster [31]. In another study examining the coherencies related to the event in patients with mild AD using visual sparse stimuli, the authors found higher OI coherence in the "delta," "theta," and "alpha" bands compared to the controls in the AD group that did not receive drug treatment. Alpha OI coherence values are higher in the medicated group compared to the drug-free AD group [32].

6. Conclusion

AD is a progressive neurocognitive disease in the elderly population. This disease is characterized by behavioral problems, cognitive impairment, delirium, and memory loss.

Most studies in AD have been done on frequency changes with EEG reactivity. When eyes are open, theta and alpha reactivity index and alpha/theta index were integrated into this study and were found as a useful approach to evaluate quantitative EEG (qEEG). EEG is advantageous compared to functional MRI or PET, which indirectly detects metabolic signals due to its noninvasive, wide availability, low cost, and direct access to neuronal signaling. Studies reveal that neuritic plaques, nodes, tangles, granulovacuolar degeneration, and the formation of amyloid angiopathy are some of the pathological variations that cause AD. Neuroprotective and symptomatic approaches such as antioxidants and neurotransmitters are effective in treating AD symptoms and delay their development. No cure can treat AD, but medications that can treat disease symptoms and delay its progression have been developed and will continue to be developed. Therefore, early diagnosis is the key in treating the disease. Advances in neuroimaging technology, cognitive neuroscience, psychopathology, neuropathology, and neurobiology lead to the discovery of AD biomarkers for early detection.

Researchers are also working on improving the accuracy of EEG-based AD diagnosis. New studies are needed to develop an algorithm in the early onset diagnosis of AD, and this will happen sometime in the future.

Acknowledgements

We would like to thank Grifolscompany for its support in publishing this section.

Conflict of interest

The authors proclaim that they have no competing interests.

Author details

Demet Ilhan Algin[1*], Demet Ozbabalık Adapinar[2] and Oguz Osman Erdinc[1]

1 Neurology Department, Eskisehir Osmangazi University, Medical Faculty, Eskisehir, Turkey

2 Neurology Department, Atlas University Medical Faculty, Istanbul, Turkey

*Address all correspondence to: demetozbabalik@gmail.com

References

[1] Cassani R, Estarellas M, San-Martin R, Fraga JF, Falk HT. Systematic Review on Resting EEG for Alzheimer's Diseases Diagnosis. 2018. p. 26

[2] World Health Organization and Alzheimer's Disease International. Dementia: A Public Health Priority. WHO; 2012. p. 112

[3] Duthey B. "Background paper 6.11: Alzheimer disease and other dementias," A Public Health Approach to Innovation. 2013. pp. 1-74

[4] Prince M, Wimo A, Guerchet M, Ali G-C, Wu Y-T, Prina M. World Alzheimer Report 2015-the Global Impact of Dementia: An Analysis of Prevalence, Incidence, Cost and Trends. Alzheimer's Disease International; 2015. p. 84

[5] Dubois B, Hampel H, Feldman HH, et al. Preclinical Alzheimer's disease: Definition, natural history, and diagnostic criteria. Alzheimer's & Dementia. 2016;**12**(3):292-323

[6] Albert MS, DeKosky ST, Dickson D, Dubois B, Feldman HH, Fox NC, et al. The diagnosis of mild cognitive impairment due to Alzheimer's disease: Recommendations from the National Institute on Aging and Alzheimer's Association Workgroup. Alzheimers Dement. 2011;**7**(3):270-279

[7] Terry RD. Neuropathological changes in Alzheimer disease. Progress in Brain Research. 1994;**101**:383-390

[8] Sarazin M, de Souza LC, Lehéricy S, Dubois B. Clinical and research diagnostic criteria for Alzheimer's disease. Neuroimaging Clinics of North America. 2012;**22**(1):23-32

[9] Sperling RA, Aisen PS, Beckett LA, et al. Toward defining the preclinical stages of Alzheimer's disease: recommendations from the National Institute on Aging-Alzheimer's Association workgroups on diagnostic guidelines for Alzheimer's disease. Alzheimers Dement. 2011;**7**(3):280-292

[10] Weiner MW, Veitch DP, Aisen PS, et al. 2014 Update of the Alzheimer's Disease Neuroimaging Initiative: A review of papers published since its inception. Alzheimers Dement. 2015;**11**(6):1-120

[11] McKhann GM, Knopman DS, Chertkow H, Hyman BT, Jack CR Jr, Kawas CH, et al. The diagnosis of dementia due to Alzheimer's disease: Recommendations from the National Institute on Aging and the Alzheimer's Association Workgroup. Alzheimers Dement. 2011;**7**(3):263-269

[12] Blennow K, de Leon MJ, Zetterberg H. Alzheimer's disease. Lancet. 2006;**368**(9533):387-403

[13] Counts ES, Ikonomovic DM, Mercado N, Vega EI, Mufson JE. Biomarkers for the early detection and progression of Alzheimer's disease. Neurotherapeutics. 2017;**14**(1):35-53

[14] Buerger K, Ewers M, Pirttila T, et al. CSF phosphorylated tau protein correlates with neocortical neurofibrillary pathology in Alzheimer's disease. Brain. 2006;**129**(11):3035-3041

[15] Seppala TT, Nerg O, Koivisto AM, et al. CSF biomarkers for Alzheimer disease correlate with cortical brain biopsy findings. Neurology. 2012;**78**(20):1568-1575

[16] Adeli H, Ghosh-Dastidar S, Dadmehr N. A spatiotemporal wavelet-chaos methodology for EEG-based diagnosis of Alzheimer's disease. Neuroscience Letters. 2008;**444**(2):190-194

[17] Ghosh-Dastidar S, Adeli H, Dadmehr N. Principal component analysis-enhanced cosine radial basis function neural network for robust epilepsy and seizure detection. IEEE Transactions on Biomedical Engineering. 2008;**55**(2):512-518

[18] de Waal H, Stam CJ, Blankenstein MA, Pij-Nenburg YA, Scheltens P, van der Flier WM. EEG abnormalities in early and late onset Alzheimer's disease, understanding heterogeneity. Journal of Neurology, Neurosurgery, and Psychiatry. 2011;**82**(1):67-71

[19] Jelic V, Johansson SE, Almkvist O, Shigeta M, Julin P, Nordberg A, et al. Quantitative electroencephalography in mild cognitive impairment, longitudinal changes and possible prediction of Alzheimer's disease. Neurobiology of Aging. 2000;**21**(4):533-540

[20] Osipova D, Ahveninen J, Jensen O, Ylikoski A, Pekkonen E. Altered generation of spontaneous oscillations in Alzheimer's disease. NeuroImage. 2005;**27**(4):835-841

[21] Babiloni C, Visser PJ, Frisoni G, De Deyn PP, Bresciani L, Jelic V, et al. Cortical sources of resting EEG rhythms in mild cognitive impairment and subjective memory complaint. Neurobiology of Aging. 2010;**31**(10):1787-1798

[22] Babiloni C, Frisoni G, Steriade M, Bresciani L, Binetti G, Del Percio C, et al. Frontal white matter volume and delta EEG sources negatively correlate in awake subjects with mild cognitive impairment and Alzheimer's disease. Clinical Neurophysiology. 2006;**117**(5):1113-1129

[23] Shute CCD, Lewis PR. The ascending cholinergic reticular system: Neocortical, olfactory, and subcortical projections. Brain. 1967;**90**:497-520

[24] Semba K. Multiple output pathways of the basal forebrain: Organization, chemical heterogeneity, and roles in vigilance. Behavioural Brain Research. 2000;**115**(2):117-141

[25] Yener GG, Güntekin B, Öniz A, Başar E. Increased frontal phase-locking of event-related theta oscillations in Alzheimer patients treated with cholinesterase inhibitors. International Journal of Psychophysiology. 2007;**64**(1):46-52

[26] Smailovic U, Koenig T, Kareholt I, Andersson T, Kramberger MG, Winblad B, et al. Quantitative EEG power and synchronization correlate with Alzheimer's disease CSF biomarkers. Neurobiology of Aging. 2018;**63**:88-95

[27] Yener GG, Güntekin B, Tülay E, Başar E. A comparative analysis of sensory visual evoked oscillations with visual cognitive event related oscillations in Alzheimer's disease. Neuroscience Letters. 2009;**462**(3):193-197

[28] Gardner WA. Unifying view of coherence in signal processing. Signal Processing. 1993;**29**:113-140

[29] Lachaux JP, Lutz A, Rudrauf D, Cosmelli D, Quyen MLV, Martinerie J, et al. Estimating the time course of coherence between single-trial brain signals, an introduction to wavelet coherence. Neurophysiologie Clinique. 2002;**32**(3):157-174

[30] Hogan MJ, Swanwick GR, Kaiser J, Rowan M, Lawlor B. Memory-related EEG power and coherence reductions in mild Alzheimer's disease. International Journal of Psychophysiology. 2003;**49**(2):147-163

[31] Rossini PM, Del Percio C, Pasqualetti P, Cassetta E, Binetti G, Dal Forno G, et al. Conversion from mild cognitive impairment to

Alzheimer's disease is predicted by sources and coherence of brain electroencephalography rhythms. Neuroscience. 2006;**143**(3):793-803

[32] Güntekin B, Saatçi E, Yener G. Decrease of evoked delta, theta and alpha coherence in Alzheimer patients during a visual oddball paradigm. Brain Research. 2008;**1235**:109-116

Chapter 6

Multi-Target-Directed Ligands in Alzheimer's Disease Therapy

Eugenie Nepovimova and Kamil Kuca

Abstract

So far, the only clinically approved drugs that are effective in Alzheimer's disease (AD) are those neurotransmitters oriented in their mode of action and focus, in particular, on the functional significance of acetylcholine or glutamate in the brain. Current AD drugs can, therefore, reduce the severity of cognitive symptoms, improve the quality of life, and stabilize the symptoms for some years, but they are not able to significantly modify the course of the disease. Complex disorders such as neurodegenerative diseases tend to result from multiple molecular abnormalities, not from a single defect. Moreover, a single target is unlikely to help in such cases because the cells can often find ways to compensate for a protein whose activity is affected by a drug. Thus, these limitations of the conventional "one-target, one-molecule" paradigm have triggered a recent shift in efforts to create drugs that hit more than one target simultaneously. The term multi-target-directed ligands (MTDLs) have been proposed to describe these hybrid molecules that are effective in treating complex diseases. Within our contribution, we would like to present general overview of MTDL design strategy in AD therapy, its positives and negatives, and finally summary of such multipotent compounds evaluated in clinical trials.

Keywords: Alzheimer's disease, therapy, multi target directed ligands, drug design, ladostigil, ANAVEX 2-73

1. Introduction

Alzheimer's disease (AD) is a progressive neurodegenerative disorder with unknown etiology. Currently, no causal treatment is available, probably due to multiple factors involved in pathophysiology of the disease. Recently, it has become clear that "one-target, one-molecule" therapy is not effective to complex diseases with multifactorial pathogenesis. Thus, novel approach, called multi-target-directed ligand (MTDL) strategy, has been developed. Hybrid compounds resulting from this drug design strategy have to be capable to act at diverse biological targets simultaneously. Discovery and subsequent launch of such multipotent drug candidates on the pharmaceutical market would greatly facilitate and improve therapeutic strategies of Alzheimer's disease.

2. Drug design history leading to multi-target-directed ligand strategy

The "one-target, one-molecule" philosophy has resulted in many approved drugs and will likely continue to be the benchmark in the time to come [1]. This paradigm has been driven by the notion that a single target's selective modulation can help create the needed extend of efficiency while simultaneously bringing down the risk of off-target side effects. On the other hand, current research has shown that the failure of such compounds is largely owed to poor safety and poor efficiency, observed in the last 10 years. It has therefore been put forward that the biology networks' intrinsic robustness and redundancy are the main culprits when it comes to highly selective drugs failing to ensure that the needed impact or result is present [2]. Furthermore, substances that focus on one target likely prove to be ineffective or insufficient when the treatment is being focused on complex illnesses, including diabetes mellitus, neurodegenerative disorders, cardiovascular diseases, and cancer that come laced with several pathogenic aspects [1].

After three decades, it seems that this approach is not effective in terms of possible success. Some of these substances only prove to be helpful to a specific set of the population [3]. When a "one-target, one-molecule" drug is not effective enough to address an illness, the next route involves several drugs administered together. Such approach is sometimes denoted as "cocktail of drugs," where multiple substances are mixed together to tackle the illness [1]. These mixtures typically contain two or more substances that come together to produce a more holistic impact [4]. This approach helps not only to increase the efficiency of the therapy but also to address and bring down the side effects – such a situation is not possible when only a single drug is being used to provide therapy. This positive situation has been observed within the treatment of several maladies, including hypertension, HIV, and cancer. However, the benefits of taking several drugs can become shaky if the patient does not comply with the regime properly. This is especially typical for situations when the illness is asymptomatic [2].

In recent times, multicomponent drugs have become more popular, where two agents or more are mixed into a single tablet, so that patient's compliance can be improved alongside the dosing schedules [2, 4]. Such combinations are called "fixed drug combinations" (FDCs). On the other hand, the problems that stem from highly complicated pharmacodynamics/pharmacokinetics necessitate formulations that have the right kind of sophistication due to the occurrence of possible drug-drug interactions, which could have a considerable impact on the costs and risks of designed FDCs [2].

Two independent scientific groups of Inestrosa and Brimijoin found out that the active site of enzyme acetylcholinesterase (AChE; E.C. 3.1.1.7) is close enough to its allosteric peripheral site and that these two sites can be spanned by one molecule at the same time. This discovery has launched rational design of novel class of therapeutic agents – dual-binding site acetylcholinesterase inhibitors (AChEIs) [5]. Inestrosa and Brimijoin in their studies demonstrated that AChE interacts through its allosteric site with amyloid peptide (Aβ) and acts thus like a pathological chaperone inducing a conformational change favoring Aβ aggregation [6, 7]. In this respect, ligands that can simultaneously interact with both sites could produce many merits comparing to active site inhibitors. Namely, such dual-binding site inhibitors considerably increase the inhibitory potential toward AChE, thus providing symptomatic relief, facilitating memory process, and, at the same time, exerting neuroprotective preventive effect [8]. Positive effects of dual-binding site inhibitors, AD's multifactorial aspect, and the routine of use of combination therapy in clinical practice prompted drug designers to pay more attention to development of more complex medicaments that in turn use dual-binding site inhibitors as an appropriate starting point [9].

Cancer, depression, neurodegenerative maladies, cardiovascular diseases, and other complex disorders typically result from several abnormalities at the molecular level, not because of a single issue. Moreover, modulation of one single target would probably not show any significance in such cases since the cells will likely find routes through which the protein can be compensated after its activity is affected by the medicine. Thus, these limitations of the conventional "one-target, one-molecule" paradigm have induced a shift in pharmaceutical companies' research to develop therapeutics that can address more than one problem. Many research groups and pharma companies now look for compounds that can address multiple issues and are even attempting to develop the so-called promiscuous drugs [3, 10]. With this new drug design strategy, two or more compounds, binding with a very high selectivity to their respective targets, are used as the starting blocks, and their structural elements are combined into a single molecule to incorporate activity at both targets. Hence, this approach normally involves the use of two or more different pharmacophoric moieties (in most cases, at least one is directly related to AChEI being a pillar of standard AD therapy) to include into a single framework [4, 10]. The term multi-target-directed ligand has been proposed to describe these hybrid molecules that could be effective in treating complex diseases [1].

3. Advantages and disadvantages of MTDLs

The use of such promiscuous drugs may provide some advantages: (i) in terms of the disease, various pathways can be effectively targeted via a single multipotent molecule, thus increasing its efficiency; (ii) drugs of a promiscuous nature do not always overactivate or suppress a network or pathway; (iii) single molecular species, although consisting of several pharmacophores, show a complex ADMET profile; (iv) drug-drug interactions' risk should be reduced; and (v) the drug regimen of the patients taking MTDLs should be greatly simplified [1, 11]. However, beside the advantages, there are also several drawbacks. A key problem linked to the use of promiscuous drugs has to do with how hard it is to optimize potencies for two different targets while using one medicine. Taking into account all the advantages and disadvantages, therapy that uses one medicine with several biological activities will prove to be inherently better than FDCs or cocktails of drugs.

4. Classification of MTDLs

Depending on the extent to which the frameworks of selective pharmacophores have been integrated, three different classes of MTDLs can be distinguished (**Figure 1**). The first class is represented by linked MTDLs, whose molecular frameworks have not been integrated but have been connected via a specific linker not found in either of the starting selective pharmacophores. Sometimes, pharmacophores in linked MTDLs contain a metabolically cleavable linker, purposely designed to exude *in vivo* two ligands that can independently interact with related targets. Such scenario could be considered as a half-way between real MTDLs and FDCs. However, in most cases, the linker is designed to be metabolically stable, yielding a single compound capable of interacting with two targets simultaneously. In particular, dual-binding site inhibitors are the best representatives of linked subclass. Fused MTDLs constitute the second class. In fused MTDLs, the frameworks are linked directly. However, medicinal chemists generally aspire to maximize the degree of framework overlap in order to design as simplest and smallest molecules as possible with favorable physicochemical properties. Therefore, it would probably not be surprising that the most common and sought after are merged MTDLs, where the frameworks are integrated by the use of commonalities in the structures of the starting compounds [2].

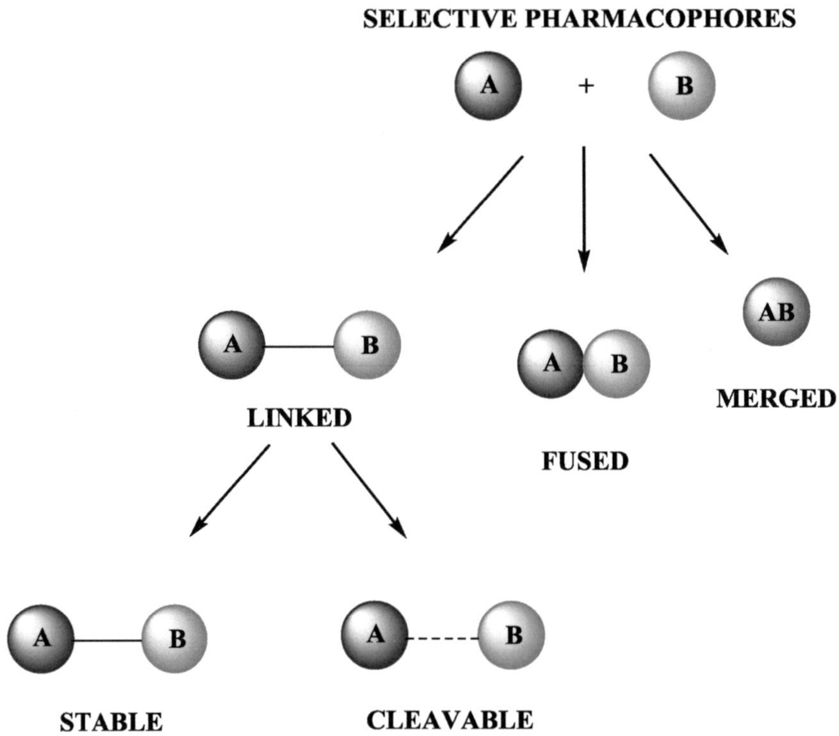

Figure 1.
Classification of MTDLs.

5. MTDLs in clinical trials

In Alzheimer's disease drug development pipeline for year 2019 issued annually by Alzheimer's and Dementia, there was no MTDL currently assessed in AD clinical trials [12]. The only drug candidate with multimodal action found within the mentioned list was ANAVEX 2-73. However, for completeness of the subchapter, we have decided to include also ladostigil as the only real representative of MTDLs ever evaluated in clinics.

Ladostigil (TV3326; **Figure 2**) is a dual cholinesterase (ChE) and brain-selective monoaminooxidase-A (MAO-A) and monoaminooxidase-B (MAO-B) inhibitor indicated for the treatment of dementia comorbid with extrapyramidal disorders and depression [13]. The design of this MTDL is based on the combination of carbamate rivastigmine and *N*-propargyl scaffold of anti-Parkinsonian drug and irreversible selective MAO-B inhibitor, rasagiline [14, 15].

Rasagiline is an irreversible inhibitor of MAO-B used as a monotherapy to treat symptoms of early Parkinson's disease (PD) or as an adjunct therapy in more advanced cases of PD [16]. Rivastigmine is a nonselective AChE and butyrylcholinesterase (BChE; E.C. 3.1.1.8) inhibitor [17]. It could be also classified as pseudo-irreversible

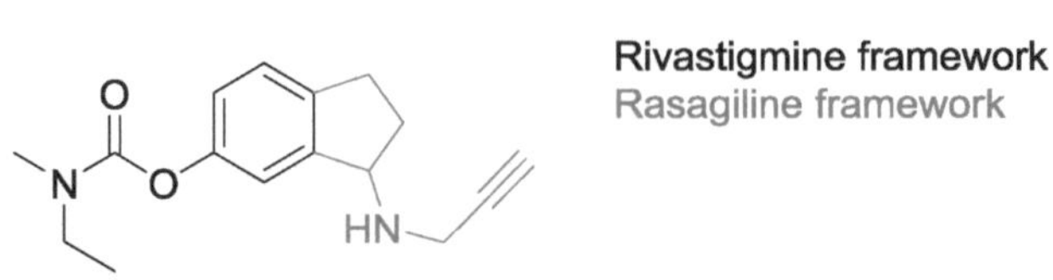

Figure 2.
Chemical structure of ladostigil.

ChE inhibitor since the duration of inhibition is longer than its elimination half-life [18]. It is indicated for the treatment of mild-to-moderate dementia associated with Alzheimer's disease type and PD [18]. Rivastigmine has also proven efficacy in decreasing psychiatric symptoms and cognitive deficits [19]. This fact together with the continued beneficial effect observed in rivastigmine-treated patients after drug withdrawal indicated disease-modifying effect [20].

In rodents, oral administration of ladostigil was shown to antagonize scopolamine-induced spatial memory impairments, pointing out that it is able to sufficiently penetrate the blood-brain barrier [21]. Apart from MAO and ChE inhibition, ladostigil has shown to possess a broad scale of neuroprotective activities against a variety of neurotoxins and neuronal cell culture models of neurodegeneration [20].

All these perspective preclinical results forwarded ladostigil to clinical evaluation. In 2011, Avraham Pharmaceuticals evaluated a 6-month trial of ladostigil in Phase II in 201 people with mild-to-moderate Alzheimer's disease. However, this trial missed its primary endpoint on the ADAS-cog11, and thus, development for Alzheimer's disease was terminated [22, 23]. In January 2012, the same company started the second Phase II study, in this case evaluating a lower dose of ladostigil for its ability to delay progression from mild cognitive impairment (MCI) to AD. This study enrolled 210 people with a clinical diagnosis of MCI. In September 2016, the company disclosed that ladostigil missed its primary endpoint in this trial as well [22, 24].

ANAVEX 2-73 (blarcamesine; **Figure 3**) is an experimental drug in Phase II clinical trial for Alzheimer's disease, Phase I for epilepsy, and preclinical trials for amyotrophic lateral sclerosis, Parkinson's disease, Rett syndrome, and stroke [25, 26]. From the pharmacological point of view, this small molecule acts as a muscarinic receptor agonist and activator of sigma-1 receptors.

Within preclinical trials, ANAVEX 2-73 alleviated scopolamine- and dizocilpine-induced learning impairments, pointing out to its antimuscarinic and neuroprotective effect mediated by NMDA receptors [27, 28]. The sigma-1 receptors are small transmembrane stress-reducing survival proteins, mainly located on the endoplasmic reticulum membrane of cells. Moreover, these receptors are known to modulate cellular processes relevant to neurodegeneration. In particular, ANAVEX 2-73 is thought to help to restore cellular balance by targeting protein misfolding, oxidative stress, mitochondrial dysfunction, inflammation, and cellular stress [29]. More recently, the effect of ANAVEX 2-73 on the main hallmarks, that is, $A\beta_{1-42}$ seeding and tau hyperphosphorylation, of Alzheimer's disease has been studied. The results of such experiment revealed that ANAVEX 2-73 significantly blocked an increase in $A\beta_{1-42}$ levels in hippocampus, suggesting that it may alleviate amyloid load in AD model. In addition, the data presented within the same study suggested that modulation of both receptors, that is, muscarinic and sigma-1, targets GSK-3β activity and that inhibiting of this kinase efficiently decreases tau hyperphosphorylation and Aβ accumulation in AD model [25].

Phase I clinical trial, assessing safety and pharmacokinetics, with ANAVEX 2-73 was successfully completed in healthy volunteers in Germany. The maximum

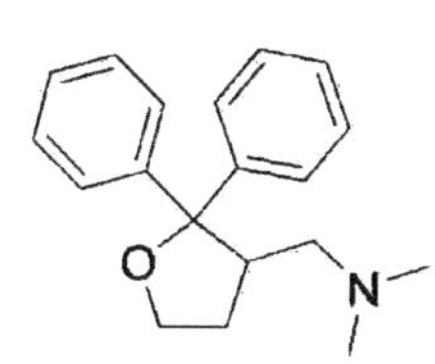

Figure 3.
Chemical structure of ANAVEX 2-73.

tolerated dose in men was determined to be 55 mg. The results of Phase II clinical trial on patients with mild-to-moderate Alzheimer's disease showed a significant association between the dosage of ANAVEX2-73 and the cognitive and function improvements [29].

6. Conclusion

While AChEI itself is an ever evolving branch of AD research, the rationale for MTDL design strategy clearly stems from the AD's multifactorial etiological basis. In a meanwhile, novel therapeutic targets continually emerge. Optimization of the therapeutic potential of dual-binding site AChEIs by adding biological activities, such as one from the arsenal against neurodegeneration, is an ongoing process for medicinal chemists. Several approaches are being deployed to design MTDLs; however, all of them use the combination of different smaller fragments of a given specific activity in a single molecule. Future work on such design strategy will involve fine tuning of pharmacokinetic and activity profiles of novel drug candidates for the purpose of modulating the selected molecular targets at the similar levels. Additionally, more clinical trials are required to prove the MTDL concept. The way ahead is not a short one; however, it is extremely possible that MTDLs could become the future treatment against AD and other similar complex multifactorial diseases, including infectious disorders, cancer, cardiovascular maladies, and so on.

Acknowledgements

This work was supported by the University of Hradec Kralove (Faculty of Science, VT2019-2021).

Conflict of interest

The authors declare no conflict of interest.

Author details

Eugenie Nepovimova and Kamil Kuca*
Department of Chemistry, Faculty of Science, University of Hradec Kralove, Hradec Kralove, Czech Republic

*Address all correspondence to: kamil.kuca@uhk.cz

References

[1] Cavalli A, Bolognesi ML, Minarini A, Rosini M, Tumiatti V, Recanatini M, et al. Multi-target-directed ligands to combat neurodegenerative diseases. Journal of Medicinal Chemistry. 2008;**51**(3):347-372

[2] Morphy R, Rankovic Z. Designing multiple ligands—Medicinal chemistry strategies and challenges. Current Pharmaceutical Design. 2009;**15**(6):587-600

[3] Frantz S. Drug discovery: Playing dirty. Nature. 2005;**437**(7061):942-943

[4] Rampa A, Belluti F, Gobbi S, Bisi A. Hybrid-based multi-target ligands for the treatment of Alzheimer's disease. Current Topics in Medicinal Chemistry. 2011;**11**(22):2716-2730

[5] Muñoz-Torrero D. Acetyl-cholinesterase inhibitors as disease-modifying therapies for Alzheimer's disease. Current Medicinal Chemistry. 2008;**15**(24):2433-2455

[6] Inestrosa NC, Alvarez A, Pérez CA, Moreno RD, Vicente M, Linker C, et al. Acetylcholinesterase accelerates assembly of amyloid-beta-peptides into Alzheimer's fibrils: Possible role of the peripheral site of the enzyme. Neuron. 1996;**16**(4):881-891

[7] Rees T, Hammond PI, Soreq H, YounkinS,BrimijoinS.Acetylcholinesterase promotes beta-amyloid plaques in cerebral cortex. Neurobiology of Aging. 2003;**24**(6):777-787

[8] Castro A, Martinez A. Peripheral and dual binding site acetylcholinesterase inhibitors: Implications in treatment of Alzheimer's disease. Mini Reviews in Medicinal Chemistry. 2001;**1**(3):267-272

[9] Bolognesi ML, Minarini A, Rosini M, Tumiatti V, Melchiorre C. From dual binding site acetylcholinesterase inhibitors to multi-target-directed ligands (MTDLs): A step forward in the treatment of Alzheimer's disease. Mini Reviews in Medicinal Chemistry. 2008;**8**(10):960-967

[10] Bolognesi ML, Rosini M, Andrisano V, Bartolini M, Minarini A, Tumiatti V, et al. MTDL design strategy in the context of Alzheimer's disease: From lipocrine to memoquin and beyond. Current Pharmaceutical Design. 2009;**15**(6):601-613

[11] Espinoza-Fonseca LM. The benefits of the multi-target approach in drug design and discovery. Bioorganic & Medicinal Chemistry. 2006;**14**(4):896-897

[12] Cummings J, Lee G, Ritter A, Sabbagh M, Zhong K. Alzheimer's disease drug development pipeline. Alzheimers & Dementia (NY). 2019;**5**: 272-293

[13] Weinreb O, Amit T, Bar-Am O, Youdim MBH. Ladostigil: A novel multimodal neuroprotective drug with cholinesterase and brain-selective monoamine oxidase inhibitory activities for Alzheimer's disease treatment. Current Drug Targets. 2012;**13**(4):483-494

[14] Weinstock M, Bejar C, Wang RH, Poltyrev T, Gross A, Finberg JP, et al. TV3326, a novel neuroprotective drug with cholinesterase and monoamine oxidase inhibitory activities for the treatment of Alzheimer's disease. Journal of Neural Transmission. Supplementum. 2000;**60**:157-169

[15] Korábečný J, Nepovimová E, Cikánková T, Špilovská K, Vašková L, Mezeiová E, et al. Newly developed drugs for Alzheimer's disease in relation to energy metabolism, cholinergic and monoaminergic neurotransmission. Neuroscience. 2018;**370**:191-206

[16] Gallagher DA, Schrag A. Impact of newer pharmacological treatments on quality of life in patients with Parkinson's disease. CNS Drugs. 2008;**22**(7):563-586

[17] Zemek F, Drtinova L, Nepovimova E, Sepsova V, Korabecny J, Klimes J, et al. Outcomes of Alzheimer's disease therapy with acetylcholinesterase inhibitors and memantine. Expert Opinion on Drug Safety. 2014;**13**(6): 759-774

[18] Dhillon S. Rivastigmine transdermal patch: A review of its use in the management of dementia of the Alzheimer's type. Drugs. 2011;**71**(9):1209-1231

[19] Farlow MR. Update on rivastigmine. The Neurologist. 2003;**9**(5):230-234

[20] Weinreb O, Amit T, Bar-Am O, Youdim MBH. A novel anti-Alzheimer's disease drug, ladostigil neuroprotective, multimodal brain-selective monoamine oxidase and cholinesterase inhibitor. International Review of Neurobiology. 2011;**100**:191-215

[21] Weinstock M, Gorodetsky E, Poltyrev T, Gross A, Sagi Y, Youdim M. A novel cholinesterase and brain-selective monoamine oxidase inhibitor for the treatment of dementia comorbid with depression and Parkinson's disease. Progress in Neuro-Psychopharmacology & Biological Psychiatry. 2003;**27**(4):555-561

[22] Ladostigil [Internet]. 2017. Dostupné z: http://www.alzforum.org/therapeutics/ladostigil

[23] Avraham closes its AD program and concentrates on the development of ladostigil to MCI, due to failure of its clinical trial [Internet]. 2017. Dostupné z: http://www.avphar.com/closing-ad-program/

[24] Clinical Data [Internet]. 2017. Dostupné z: http://www.avphar.com/ladostigil/clinical-data/

[25] Villard V, Espallergues J, Keller E, Vamvakides A, Maurice T. Anti-amnesic and neuroprotective potentials of the mixed muscarinic receptor/sigma 1 (σ1) ligand ANAVEX2-73, a novel aminotetrahydrofuran derivative. Journal of Psychopharmacology Oxford England. 2011;**25**(8):1101-1117

[26] Blarcamesine. Anavex Life Sciences. AdisInsight [Internet]. Dostupné z: https://adisinsight.springer.com/drugs/800033840

[27] Maurice T, Hiramatsu M, Itoh J, Kameyama T, Hasegawa T, Nabeshima T. Behavioral evidence for a modulating role of sigma ligands in memory processes. I. Attenuation of dizocilpine (MK-801)-induced amnesia. Brain Research. 1994;**647**(1):44-56

[28] Senda T, Matsuno K, Kobayashi T, Mita S. Reduction of the scopolamine-induced impairment of passive-avoidance performance by sigma receptor agonist in mice. Physiology & Behavior. 1997;**61**(2):257-264

[29] PhD EM. Anavex 2-73 [Internet]. Alzheimer's News Today. 2017. Dostupné z: https://alzheimersnewstoday.com/anavex-2-73/

Section 3

Polyglutamine Pathology, Huntington's Disease and Stem Cell Approach in Therapy

Chapter 7

Molecular Mechanisms of Polyglutamine Pathology and Lessons Learned from Huntington's Disease

Nagehan Ersoy Tunalı

Abstract

Identification of polymorphic repeating units on DNA as a cause of many neurological disorders has introduced a new concept in molecular biology: Dynamic mutations. Many of the identified dynamic mutations involve expansion of trinucleotide repeats within disease genes. Nine neurodegenerative disorders are currently known to be caused by expanding CAG trinucleotide repeats. These are Huntington's Disease (HD), Dentato-Rubral Pallidoluysian Atrophy (DRPLA), Spinal and Bulbar Muscular Atrophy (SBMA), and Spinocerebellar Ataxia (SCA) Type 1, 2, 3, 6, 7 and 17. All are inherited in an autosomal dominant fashion except for SBMA, which is X-linked recessive. In all polyQ diseases, the disease mutation involves an increase in the number of CAG repeats within the coding regions of the respective genes. Since CAG triplets encode glutamine in the proteins, diseases caused by CAG repeat expansions are known as "Polyglutamine (polyQ) Diseases". PolyQ diseases share certain clinical, neuropathological and molecular findings. The most widely studied polyQ disease is HD. In HD and other polyQ diseases, conformational change in the mutant protein causes abnormal folding and proteolysis of the protein, leading to the formation of a toxic polyQ fragment, which aggregates and causes neuronal dysfunction and selective neuronal death in the brain.

Keywords: polyglutamine diseases, trinucleotide repeats, Huntington's disease, CAG expansion, neuronal death

1. PolyQ diseases

1.1 Clinical and neuropathological characteristics of PolyQ diseases

Despite a wide spectrum of clinical presentations, all polyQ diseases are characterized by late onset and progressive neurodegeneration, involving selective neuron death. Clinical symptoms generally begin in midlife, although they can also manifest earlier. In all cases, age of onset is inversely related to the CAG repeat size in respective genes. Larger CAG repeat tracts were found to be associated with earlier disease onset, severe phenotype and rapid progression [1]. The expanded repeat tracts are prone to changes in length during intergenerational transmission. This results in earlier disease onset in the later generations, known as anticipation.

The pathology of polyQ diseases involves selective neuronal degeneration mostly in the central nervous system (CNS). PolyQ disease loci, polyQ proteins and repeat sizes are shown in **Table 1**, and the clinical and neuropathological characteristics of polyQ diseases are listed in **Table 2** [2].

1.2 Genotype-phenotype correlations in polyQ diseases

CAG repeat sizes on polyQ alleles are generally categorized in three main groups, being normal, intermediate and pathogenic. Alleles with repeat numbers in the normal range are not associated with disease state. Intermediate alleles usually do not cause disease, but have a great tendency to increase in number upon vertical transmission and may cause disease in the next generation. Alleles having repeat numbers in the pathological range definitely cause the disease in a normal life span. Composition of the repeat tract is important in determining the disease state, as well as the size of the repeats. In SCA1 and SCA2, CAG repeat tracts on normal alleles are usually interrupted with other triplets, increasing the stability of DNA. However, disease alleles contain uninterrupted, pure CAG repeats. SCA1 normal alleles are almost always interrupted with one to three CAT repeats, and the disease causing expanded alleles consist of perfect CAG repeat tracts, with one reported exception of an expanded allele (58 repeats) interrupted by two CAT triplets [3]. Later onset of disease than expected in this patient suggests that the sequence composition of the repeat tract may be an important determinant in SCA1 disease manifestation. SCA2 normal alleles contain one to three CAA interruptions, with only two reported exceptions of pure 14 and 29 CAG repeats [4].

1.3 Mechanisms of polyQ pathogenesis

Although polyQ proteins are expressed widely in all cell and tissue types, each disease is characterized by selective neuron degeneration. The molecular mechanism of neurodegeneration is not clear yet, but the properties of mutant polyQ proteins provide important clues, and it is very likely that all the diseases in this group share similar mechanisms of pathogenesis. The very first effect of the repeat expansion mutation is proved to be the conformational change of the mutant protein. The new conformation of the mutant polyQ proteins was shown to confer a novel deleterious function [5].

Disease	Locus	Protein	Protein size (kDa)	CAG	Repeat	Ranges
				Normal	Intermediate	Pathogenic
HD	4p16	Huntingtin	348	6–35	29–39	36–250
DRPLA	12p13	Atrophin-1	190	3–35	_	49–88
SBMA	Xq11-q12	Androgen Receptor	99	11–34	_	38–62
SCA 1	6p23	Ataxin-1	87	6–44	39–44	39–83
SCA 2	12q24.1	Ataxin-2	150	15–31	32–33	34–200
SCA 3	14q32.1	Ataxin-3	48	12–41	_	55–84
SCA 6	19p13	α_{1A}-Ca^{+2} Channel	280	4–17	_	20–33
SCA 7	3p14-21.1	Ataxin -7	96	4–35	28–35	37–306
SCA 17	6p27	TBP	42	25–42	43–46	45–63

Table 1.
PolyQ diseases.

Disease	Clinical findings	Neuropathology
HD	Involuntary choreic movements, cognitive and emotional disturbances, dementia	Cortex, basal ganglia and striatum
DRPLA	Adults: ataxia, choreathetosis, dementia Childhood: mental retardation, behavioral disturbances, myoclonus and epilepsy	Dentatorubral and pallidoluysian systems, basal ganglia, cerebellum
SBMA	Walking disability, muscle cramps, decreased deep tendon reflexes, dysarthria and dysphagia, afixation, pneumonia	Anterior horn cells in spinal cord and dorsal ganglia
SCA 1	Universal gait and limb ataxia, dysarthria, nystagmus, mild optic atrophy, hypertonia (early), hypotonia (late), decreased deep tendon reflexes, dysphagia, difficulties in breathing, extrapyramidal findings	Purkinje cells, dentate inferior olive, cranial nerve nuclei, substantia nigra, putamen, pallidum, subthalamic nucleus
SCA 2	Near universal gait and limb ataxia, dysarthria, abnormal eye movements, neuropathy, chorea, dystonia, dementia	Purkinje cells, inferior olive, pontocerebellar nuclei, substantia nigra, striatum, Clarke's column of the spinal cord, demyelination of posterior columns, cerebral cortex, spinocerebellar tracts
SCA3	Type 1: early onset, dystonia and rigidity Type 2: cerebellar and pyramidal signs Type 3: late onset, peripheral neuropathy, cerebellar signs Type 4 : parkinsonism	Globus pallidus, subthalamic nucleus, substantia nigra, dentate nucleus, pontine and cranial nerve nuclei, spinal neurons, peripheral neuropathy
SCA 6	Ophtalmoplegia, spasticity, peripheral neuropathy, dysphagia, parkinsonism, balance problems	Loss of Purkinje and granular cells, neuron death in dentate nucleus and inferior olive, atrophy in brain stem
SCA 7	Visual loss, gait and limb ataxia, dysarthria, widespread pyramidal findings, decreased vibration sense, dysphagia, hearing impairment	Retina, cerebellar Purkinje and granule cells, dentate, inferior olive, subthalamic nucleus and spinal motor neurons
SCA 17	Gait and limb ataxia, dementia, parkinsonism, chorea or dystonia	Small neurons in caudate nucleus and putamen, Purkinje cells, thalamus, frontal and temporal cortex

Table 2.
Clinical and neuropathological findings in PolyQ diseases.

Mutant polyQ proteins are cleaved by proteases, aggregate, and form inclusions in the cells. The polyQ aggregates are ubiquitinated and recruite many proteins to the aggregates, like transcription factors (TFs), chaperons, and proteasomes. The exact protein context could influence the differences in areas of neurodegeneration. Mutant proteins may lead to cell death by causing changes in protein interactions, transcriptional dysregulation and dysfunction of the ubiquitin proteasome system (UPP). On the other hand, it is also possible that partial loss of the normal functions of proteins may be contributing to disease pathogenesis [6]. So, gain and loss of function mechanisms could have convergent effects in polyQ-mediated neurotoxicity.

2. Huntington's disease

2.1 Epidemiology and clinical correlates

The first definitive description of HD was presented in 1872 by Dr. George Huntington, in his article titled "On Chorea" [7]. This article pinpoints the important essential features of the disease; its hereditary course and its manifestation in adult life. This first full description of the disease awakened the HD research, and studies concerning the origin and prevalence of the disease have started. It has been cleared that the gene originated in Northern Europe, with a prevalence of 5–10 affected people per 100 000 among individuals of European descent. Apart from Finland, there is a uniform prevalence of HD throughout Europe. The prevalence of HD in Finland is lower than that of other Northern European countries, which can be partly explained by the lower frequency of htt haplogroup A on chromosome 4 among the Finnish population.

HD is a chronic and progressive neurodegenerative disorder of the CNS, inherited in an autosomal dominant manner. The characteristic clinical features include motor, cognitive and behavioural abnormalities. HD is regarded as an adult-onset disease since the first signs appear in the third to fifth decade of life. However, the age at onset (AO) follows a normal distribution, showing a peak around the fourth decade, with some patients manifesting the disease before 20 (Juvenile HD, 5–10 per cent of HD cases) or after 60 years of age (~20 per cent of HD cases). The illness lasts for about 15–20 years. The clinical course of HD involve three basic abnormalities: Motor dysfunction, behavioural disturbances and cognitive decline. Motor abnormalities involve involuntary movements in the extremities and progress into jerky movements. The severity of involuntary movements, known as chorea, increases progressively during the initial years of the illness, and is later replaced by bradykinesia and rigidity. In the disease course, patients also develop dysarthria, dysphagia, balance problems, and incoordination. Later on rigidity dominates, which may leave the patient bed-bound or confined to a wheelchair. In juvenile HD (JHD) patients, rigidity is more common than chorea. Behavioural abnormalities usually precede the motor symptoms, including depression, anxiety, and changes in personality, however they are usually unnoticed. Suicide, the third most common cause of death among HD patients, is more common than in the general population. Through the late stages of HD, patients develop dementia, characterized by inefficient use of memory and impairment of executive functions [8].

2.2 Neuropathology of HD

The neuropathology of HD is restricted to the brain, selective loss of neurons within the striatum being the predominant hallmark. Medium sized, spiny GABA-ergic striatal output neurons are lost up to 80 per cent. Neuronal loss in HD patients begins early in life, before the manifestation of motor symptoms. At the time of motor onset of disease, cortical grey matter, subcortical white matter, and about 30 per cent of caudate neurons are already lost (**Figure 1**). These all account for loss of brain weight by 20 to 30 per cent less than normal [9]. The neuronal intranuclear inclusions (NII) found in the brain are accepted as a neuropathological marker of HD. Huntingtin inclusions were shown in the cortex and striatum of transgenic HD mice, and post-mortem HD brains [10]. Gamma Amino Butyric Acid (GABA), acetylcholine and dopamine neurotransmitters were found to be decreased in the diseased basal ganglia. Also glutamic acid decarboxylase (GAD) levels, the enzyme involved in GABA biosynthesis, is found to be reduced in the caudate, putamen and globus pallidus.

2.3 Molecular genetics of HD

2.3.1 The HD gene structure

In 1993, human HD gene was localized to chromosome 4p16.3 by positional cloning approach [11]. The HD gene, called IT-15, consists of 67 exons spanning 180 kb of DNA (**Figure 1**). The $(CAG)_n$ repeat is located in Exon 1, 17 codons downstream the ATG start codon, and encodes a highly polymorphic and unstable segment of

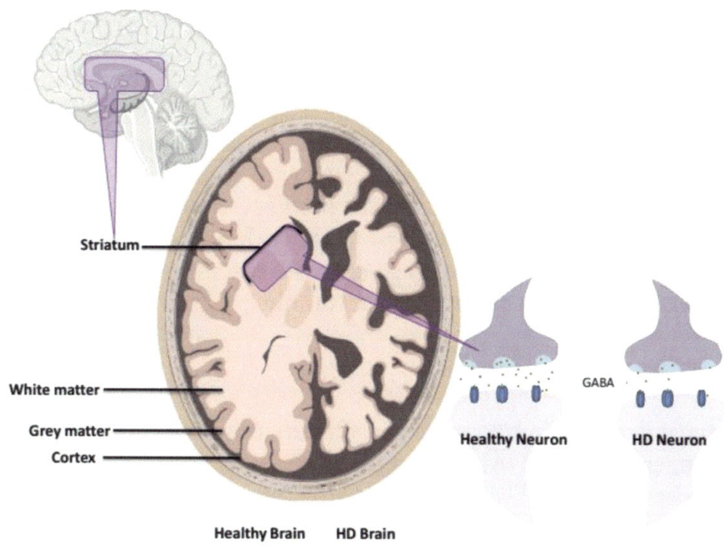

Figure 1.
Neuropathological changes in the HD brain.

glutamines. The repeat tract varies between 6–35 CAGs in healthy individuals and 36–250 CAGs in HD patients. Adjacent to $(CAG)_n$ repeats, there is a stretch of proline encoding CCG repeats, which is slightly polymorphic (6–12 repeats) and stably transmitted [12]. Most healthy chromosomes and the majority of mutant chromosomes contain seven CCG repeats. In Exon 58, there is a rare codon-loss (GAG, glutamate) polymorphism (Δ2642), which occurs in 5% of healthy and 24–38% of HD chromosomes [13]. The human HD gene is highly conserved across a wide range of species like mouse, rat, fugu, zebrafish, and pig [3, 14, 15].

2.3.2 The HD mutation

The mutation causing HD is the expansion of the CAG repeat tract in the first exon of the HD gene [11]. Healthy chromosomes contain 6–35 CAGs, and HD chromosomes possess 36–250 units [16]. The CAG repeats in the HD gene are highly unstable, resulting in expansions or contractions upon transmission to the next generation. The CAG repeat tract was shown to be unstable in 80% of the transmissions. The size and direction of the instability depend on the sex of the affected parent. In maternal transmissions, nearly equal numbers of expansions and contractions are seen, and shifts range from one to three repeats in size. In contrast, paternal transmissions are more frequently expansions. In addition to meiotic instability, a modest degree of instability was shown within and between somatic tissues of HD patients. In the brain, instability was observed in the caudate and putamen; in non-CNS tissues, most instability was observed in the liver and kidney. Three general mechanisms can be proposed to account for repeat instability: Slippage during DNA replication, misalignment with subsequent excision repair, and unequal crossover and recombination. Slippage-mediated length change during DNA replication better explains the instability in repeat size in HD.

2.3.3 Genotype-phenotype relations

There is a strong inverse correlation between age of onset (AO) and expanded CAG repeat length. The length of the expanded CAG repeat accounts for about 70%

of the variation in AO, however, repeat size alone should not be used to predict AO [16]. The second modifying factor of AO is the sex-of-parent effect, which accounts for 2–5% of the variation. Juvenile HD patients more likely inherit the disease from their fathers, and patients with late AO more frequently inherit the disease from their affected mothers [16]. The remaining variation in AO may partly be explained by environmental effects, however, studies suggest a strong genetic component, which implies that there are other genes that modify AO in HD. New mutations, resulting in de novo disease presentation have been described in HD. Higher normal repeats may expand into the pathological range and may cause disease in the next generation, leading to a new mutation in the family.

2.3.4 Huntingtin mRNA and protein

IT-15 gene is expressed ubiquitously in all human tissues in the form of two major messenger RNA (mRNA) transcripts of 13.6 kb and 10.3 kb in length, which differ in the size of the 3' UTR due to differential polyadenylation [17]. HD mRNA is expressed in both neural and non-neural tissues with high levels of expression in brain and testes [18].

The HD gene encodes a protein of 3144 amino acids with a molecular mass of 348 kDa, termed huntingtin (htt). The polyQ tract starts at residue 18 and is followed by a stretch of prolines. Protein studies also indicate ubiquitous expression of htt in various cells and tissues throughout the development and in the adult. In HD patients, normal and mutant huntingtin have a similar distribution and expression pattern [17, 18].

Huntingtin has no structural homology with other proteins, which makes the determination of its normal function difficult. The high degree of conservation across species suggests that the normal function of htt is essential. Studies of mice with targeted mutations that reduce the levels of htt to zero to 50 per cent reveal that htt also plays a critical role in embryogenesis, during brain development. Reduced levels of htt lead to perinatal lethality and abnormalities in the head region, and significantly reduced levels produce a more severe phenotype, including abnormalities in skin, placement of the ear, and excencephaly. In addition, conditional knock-out mice develop a neurodegenerative disease [19]. HD cell models revealed that the wild type (wt) protein partially protects cells from mutant htt. Htt may also be important for cell survival through growth factor (GF) stimulation, as brain-derived neurotrophic factor-rescued cells expressing mutant htt [20]. In the neuron, htt is found throughout the cell body, and in axons, dendrites, and perikarya. Its association with microtubules and vesicles [21] has suggested a role in intracellular trafficking or neurotransmission, and retrograde transport. Association of htt with the cytoskeleton and cytosolic membrane suggests a role in normal cytoskeletal function [22]. Htt is also found in cytoplasmic inclusions in Alzheimer's Disease (AD) and Parkinson's Disease, which are mostly made up of cytoskeletal proteins. The presence of htt also in the nucleus could indicate that it may be involved in nuclear processes such as transcription, replication, RNA splicing, mRNA transport, and nuclear organization. Huntingtin has no known homologies to any other protein, but it contains a few known sequence motifs with defined functions. Several proteins that interact directly with htt may give clues in understanding its possible functions. Based on their known functions, htt-interacting proteins can be grouped as proteins that are involved in gene transcription, intracellular signaling, trafficking, endocytosis or metabolism [23]. Analysis of the htt-interactors reveal that htt might function as a scaffold, controlling the proteins for signaling processes and intracellular transport [24].

2.4 Molecular pathology in HD

The general flow of the molecular pathology in HD is summarized in **Figure 2**. It starts with gain of toxic function together with loss of normal htt upon conformational change of the protein. The mutant protein aggregates and becomes more prone to proteolysis and the toxic htt fragment may interfere with transcription, leading to neuronal dysfuntion and selective neuronal death.

2.4.1 Gain and loss of function of Huntingtin

The general flow of the molecular pathology in HD is summarized in **Figure 2**. The molecular mechanism underlying polyQ pathogenesis has first been explained by toxic gain of function (GOF) of the mutant proteins. However, later findings strongly addressed loss of function of the normal proteins as a contributor to the disease process. In a mouse model, 146 CAG repeats were inserted into the HPRT gene, which is not involved in any CAG repeat disorder, in order to prove the gain of function mechanism. This mutant mice produced a polyQ expanded form of the HPRT protein and developed a late-onset neurological phenotype that resulted in death [5]. So, it is widely accepted that the polyQ mutations act by introducing a novel deleterious function to the mutant proteins. In humans, heterozygous inactivation of htt by disrupting the HD gene does not result in HD phenotype [25]. In addition, mice that have only one functioning Hdh gene do not show any features of the disease [26]. Although an expanded CAG repeat could play a major role in the disease, the possibility of a dysfunction of the wt protein in HD cannot be ruled out. These findings suggest that the toxic effect of mutant htt might lie in sequestration of normal htt or of its functions [27].

2.4.2 Conformational change of the mutant Huntingtin

The baseline of the pathogenic mechanism causing HD appears to be the unusual conformation adopted by the mutant htt protein as a result of the expanded

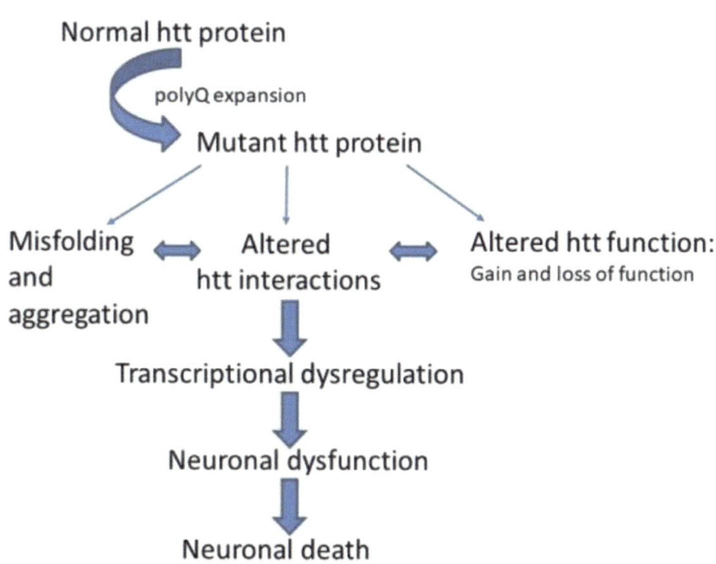

Figure 2.
Molecular pathology of HD.

polyQ segment. In a short protein fragment, the expanded polyQ tract facilitates aggregation, via conversion to an insoluble amyloid sheet structure [27]. Such a difference in the protein structure may lead to a change in the usual interactions of the protein and also may lead to abnormal interactions with other cellular factors. In addition, the mutant protein with an expanded polyQ tract may have effects on the function of the wild type protein. Two non-mutually exclusive mechanisms have been proposed to explain the aberrant conformation and subsequent aggregation of the mutant htt: Polar zipper and transglutaminase hypotheses. The polar zipper model states that the normal protein conformation is destabilized due to the presence of the expanded polyQ tract, and insolubleβ -pleated sheets may form and aggregate, by linkingβ -strands together via hydrogen bonding, forming "polar zipper" structures [28]. The transglutaminase hypothesis states that, mutant htt aggregation could be a result of the transglutaminase activity, which are normally involved in crosslinking of glutamine residues in different proteins. Huntingtin is a substrate of transglutaminase in vitro, and the rate of the reaction increases with the length of the polyQ tract [29]. According to these results, it can be hypothesized that, expanded polyQ stretch may result in increased crosslinking between mutant htt and other proteins, including itself, which may lead to aggregation.

2.4.3 Mutant protein aggregation

Transgenic mouse models of HD, expressing Exon 1 of the human HD gene with various CAG repeats numbers under the control of the human htt promoter, were established. These models served as a major step towards understanding the molecular pathology of HD. Mice expressing 18 CAG repeats developed normally and remained healthy. By contrast, mice that expressed 113 to 156 CAG repeats demonstrated progressive neurological symptoms and developed intraneuronal aggregates [21, 30]. Similar aggregates have been identified in post-mortem human cortical and striatal neurons and dystrophic neurites of HD brains [10]. Although NII occur in areas of pathology, their distribution does not correlate with the regions of neurodegeneration. In HD brains, inclusions contain truncated fragments of the mutant htt, which are recognized only by antibodies to the N-terminal region of the htt. The intranuclear inclusions are spherical or elliptical, larger than the nucleoli, and are not isolated with a membrane. Electron microscopy reveals that the inclusions contain a mixture of granules, filaments and fibrils. Intranuclear aggregates are accepted as a common pathological marker for polyQ diseases, since similar structures are seen in all polyQ diseased brains. Since the inclusions are not isolated with a membrane, they can be regarded as membrane-less compartments or organelles. The membrane-less structures, in general, are important for various essential functions in both the cytoplasm and the nucleus. They are formed through a phase separation process of RNA and protein molecules and are known to be responsive to the changes in the cellular environment. These structures are also dynamic, such that they can sequester or release proteins and RNA molecules, thereby affecting cellular stress response and neurodegenerative processes [31]. In this context, nuclear inclusions in HD should not be regarded as sole aggregates of mutant htt, but rather as a potential sink organelle for various RNA and proteins which possibly change the interactions of mutant htt and having deterministic roles in the fate of neurons with these inclusions and the neurodegenerative process in general.

Although accepted as a main pathological marker, the importance and function of the inclusions in cell culture models and HD brains are still not clear. Inclusions can be the primary cause of neuron loss, they can be beneficial by isolating the mutant protein from the rest of the cell, or just epiphenomenon. Since they appear before the disease symptoms in the transgenic mice, a causal role has been suggested [30]. In addition, inclusions well correlate with the size of the CAG repeats and susceptibility to cell death [32, 33]. Reduction of inclusions using heat shock protein HDJ-1 decreases cell death *in vitro* [34].

2.4.4 Proteolysis

Proteolysis of htt by caspases and calpains has been shown in several studies using cell culture, animal models and post-mortem analyses [35]. The toxic fragment hypothesis suggests that, the pathological mechanism of HD may rely on the production of a toxic fragment containing the polyQ tract. The basal caspase activity may be sufficient to generate small amounts of cleavage products. If this cleavage products are toxic to neurons, then accumulation would put further stress to the cell, resulting in additional caspase activation in a positive feedback loop, and eventual cell death [36]. It is possible that over the life span of the affected individual, sufficient amounts of toxic polyQ fragments may be produced from this basal activity, pushing the balance toward cell death and neurodegeneration. The model for the role of caspases suggests two major stages. First, truncated htt fragments containing the expanded polyQ tract were produced by caspases (e.g. caspase-3, caspase-6), which can be considered as a rate-limiting step. Then, additional caspase activity (e.g. as caspase-8) can be provoked that may activate the caspases (e.g. caspase-3) further, which may eventually result in cell death.

2.4.5 Role of chaperones and proteasomes

Proteins with long polyQ tracts have altered conformation and are usually misfolded. Chaperone proteins help in the folding of proteins. Several heat shock proteins (HSP) function as modulators of protein folding, thereby prevent misfolding and aggregation [37]. It was shown that HSP-40 and HSP-70 are sequestered in htt Exon 1 aggregates in cell models [38]. It is possible that redistribution into aggregates could deplete chaperones in the cells, preventing them to perform their functions.

Mutant polyQ protein aggregates were found to be ubiquitinated and associated with the proteasome apparatus. Cells tag misfolded proteins with ubiquitin, which directs them to proteasomes for degradation. In their abnormal conformations, mutant polyQ proteins might have a restricted entry into the proteolytic chamber or they might be incompletely degraded, causing jamming of the proteasomes. The depletion of proteasomal activity might lead to a build-up of many proteins normally cleared by proteasomes. Degradation of short-lived proteins is the major function of the proteasomes. The concentrations of some of these proteins, for example transcription factos, should be under strict control, since they are critical regulators of cellular homeostasis. If the proteasomal activity is impaired, the levels of short-lived proteins will rise abnormally, leading to cellular toxicity [39, 40].

2.4.6 Aggregates, nuclear localization and toxicity

Subcellular localization of the mutant polyQ proteins may be a more important determinant of toxicity, rather than the formation of aggregates. Although there is cytoplasmic pathology, many studies draw attention to the nucleus as the major site of pathogenesis. Transgenic mice, expressing expanded polyQ proteins with mutant nuclear localization signal (NLS) do not show disease pathology, and NLS-inserted polyQ proteins cause more toxicity in the cells. In addition, htt, being a cytoplasmic protein, was found in the nucleus when mutated. These findings support the hypothesis that nuclear localization of mutant polyQ proteins have an important role in disease pathogenesis [41]. Studies questioning aggregate toxicity and nuclear localization resulted in very important findings. When Q20 and Q42 peptides were subjected to cold shock, they formed fibrillar aggregates in the cells. When NLS was added to these peptides, aggregates entered into the nucleus, and both normal and mutated peptide aggregates resulted in cell death. However, cytoplasmic aggregates without NLS did not cause toxicity. Sixty five per cent of the cells with nuclear Q42 aggregates exhibited cell death in 24 hours. According to these findings, subcellular localization of the aggregates, rather than the length of the polyQ stretch seems to be more important. When NLS is added to amyloid fibril forming bacterial CspB-1 cold shock protein, aggregates are formed in the nucleus, but are not toxic. This proves that the polyQ tract itself is responsible for aggregate toxicity. Aggregate formation requires a critical polyQ concentration, and this can explain the late disease onset and the negative correlation between the repeat length and AO. Proteins with polyQ repeats in the normal range are also shown to form fibrillar aggregates *in vitro*. However, proteins with normal numbers of repeats require a higher threshold concentration for protein aggregation, and the aggregate formation process is very slow, which makes this event impossible in a normal life span [33, 34, 41].

2.4.7 Transcriptional dysregulation

Cleavage and subsequent nuclear localization of polyQ proteins may result in changes in nuclear functions, like nuclear protein turnover, transcription, and RNA processing, through interactions with various nuclear factors. The most widely studied mechanism among them is the transcriptional dysregulation. One hypothesis concerning transcriptional dysregulation is that polyQ proteins might normally interact with proteins in transcription complexes, and interactions might become aberrant when the polyQ is expanded [42]. Furthermore, mutant polyQ proteins can sequester other proteins containing polyQ stretches, like several transcription factors. Therefore, polyQ toxicity may arise from decreased availability of some transcription factors, resulting in abnormalities in the regulation of transcription. Htt was found to interact with proteins involved in transcriptional regulation, including transcriptional coactivators and corepressors. Mutant htt may be toxic through binding and depleting some of these factors. The most important TFs that are thought to be involved in HD pathogenesis are, CRE-binding protein (CREBP), p53, C-terminal binding protein (CtBP), TAFII 130 and Sp1 [43, 44].

2.4.8 Neuronal dysfunction and selective death in HD

The early disease process involves neuronal dysfunction rather than cell death, and in late stages apoptotic type of cell death occurs. Biochemical and immunohistochemical studies show N-terminal htt fragments in brain tissues from affected HD patients and not from controls. Also, increased levels of DNA strand breaks in HD patient brains imply an apoptotic mechanism [10]. Although the mutated proteins are expressed in many cell types [18], a specific pattern of neuronal degeneration occurs in each polyQ disease [45]. The selective vulnerability of striatal and cortical neurons in HD can not be explained by the level of htt expression, since other regions of the CNS express htt at the same level, but are not affected in the disease. Interactions of the polyQ containing proteins in specific cell types, sequestration of some tissue-specific transcription factors, or somatic increases in mutation size in the affected brain regions may provide an explanation. It is also possible that mutant proteins undergo cell type-specific proteolysis. Tissue-specific proteolysis can occur in two ways: Either the mutant proteins are processed with tissue specific proteases, or the mutant protein in its new conformation becomes susceptible to different proteases. In fact, tissue-specific proteolysis has been demonstrated in one study, in which proteolysis specific to striatum and cortex was shown, without any differences between healthy and HD brain [46]. No striatum specific htt interactor has been identified yet in order to suggest a tissue-specific interaction of htt, but striatum-specific transcriptional regulators can be more sensitive to htt dysfunction, causing transcriptional dysregulation. On the other hand, N-terminal htt fragments accumulate in striatal neurons and their axonal processes in HD transgenic mice. This finding supports the idea that mutant htt is proteolysed specifically and aggregates selectively in striatum [6].

Acknowledgements

I would like to thank my PhD student, Ezgi Keske, for the help in drawing **Figure 1**.

Conflict of interest

I have no conflict of interests.

Author details

Nagehan Ersoy Tunalı
Department of Molecular Biology and Genetics, İstanbul Medeniyet University, İstanbul, Turkey

*Address all correspondence to: nagehan.ersoy@medeniyet.edu.tr

References

[1] Klockgether T, Evert B. Genes involved in hereditary ataxias. Trends in Neurosciences. 1998;**21**(9):413-418

[2] Schöls L, Bauer P, Schmidt T, Schulte T, Riess O. Autosomal dominant cerebellar ataxias: clinical features, genetics, and pathogenesis. The Lancet Neurology. 2004;**3**(5):291-304

[3] Matsuyama Z, Izumi Y, Kameyama M, Kawakami H, Nakamura S. The effect of CAT trinucleotide interruptions on the age at onset of spinocerebellar ataxia type 1 (SCA1). Journal of Medical Genetics. 1999;**36**(7):546-548

[4] Saleem Q, Choudhry S, Mukerji M, Bashyam L, Padma MV, Chakravarthy A, et al. Molecular analysis of autosomal dominant hereditary ataxias in the Indian population: high frequency of SCA2 and evidence for a common founder mutation. Human Genetics. 2000;**106**(2):179-187

[5] Ordway JM, Tallaksen-Greene S, Gutekunst C-A, Bernstein EM, Cearley JA, Wiener HW, et al. Ectopically Expressed CAG Repeats Cause Intranuclear Inclusions and a Progressive Late Onset Neurological Phenotype in the Mouse. Cell. 1997;**91**(6):753-763

[6] Cattaneo E, Rigamonti D, Goffredo D, Zuccato C, Squitieri F, Spione S. Loss of normal huntingtin function: new developments in Huntington's disease research. Trends in Neurosciences. 2001;**24**(3):182-188

[7] Huntington G. On Chorea. Medical and Surgical Reporter. 1972;**26**:320-321

[8] Craufurd D. Huntington's disease. Prenatal Diagnosis. 1996;**16**(13):1237-1245

[9] Monte SM, Vonsattel JP, Richardson EP. Morphometric Demonstration of Atrophic Changes in the Cerebral Cortex, White Matter, and Neostriatum in Huntington's Disease. Journal of Neuropathology & Experimental Neurology. 1988;**47**(5):516-525

[10] DiFiglia M, Sapp E, Chase KO, Davies SW, Bates GP, Vonsattel JP, et al. Aggregation of Huntingtin in Neuronal Intranuclear Inclusions and Dystrophic Neurites in Brain. Science. 1997;**277**(5334):1990-1993

[11] MacDonald M, Ambrose CM, Duyao MP, Myers RH, Lin C, Srinidhi L, et al. A novel gene containing a trinucleotide repeat that is expanded and unstable on Huntington's disease chromosomes. Cell. 1993;**72**(6):971-983

[12] Lin B, Nasir J, Kalchman MA, Mcdonald H, Zeisler J, Goldberg YP, et al. Structural analysis of the 5′ region of mouse and human huntington disease genes reveals conservation of putative promoter region and di- and trinucleotide polymorphisms. Genomics. 1995;**25**(3):707-715

[13] MacDonald ME, Novelletto A, Lin C, Tagle D, Barnes G, Bates G, et al. The Huntington's disease candidate region exhibits many different haplotypes. Nature Genetics. 1992;**1**(2):99-103

[14] Li Z, Karlovich CA, Fish MP, Scott MP, Myers RM. A Putative Drosophila Homolog of the Huntington's Disease Gene. Human Molecular Genetics. 1999;**8**(9):1807-1815

[15] Strong TV, Tagle DA, Valdes JM, Elmer LW, Boehm K, Swaroop M, et al. Widespread expression of the human and rat Huntington's disease gene in brain and nonneural tissues. Nature Genetics. 1993;**5**(3):259-265

[16] Rubinsztein DC, Leggo J, Coles R, Almqvist E, Biancalana V, Cassiman JJ,

et al. Phenotypic Characterization of Individuals with 30-40 CAG Repeats in the Huntington Disease (HD) Gene Reveals HD Cases with 36 Repeats and Apparently Normal Elderly Individuals with 36-39 Repeats. American Journal of Human Genetics. 1996;**59**(1):16-22

[17] Trottier Y, Devys D, Imbert G, Saudou F, An I, Lutz Y, et al. Cellular localization of the Huntington's disease protein and discrimination of the normal and mutated form. Nature Genetics. 1995;**10**(1):104-110

[18] Sharp AH, Loev SJ, Schilling G, Li SH, Li XJ, Bao J, et al. Widespread expression of Huntington's disease gene (IT15) protein product. Neuron. 1995;**14**(5):1065-1074

[19] Dragatsis I, Levine MS, Zeitlin S. Inactivation of Hdh in the brain and testis results in progressive neurodegeneration and sterility in mice. Nature Genetics. 2000;**26**(3):300-306

[20] Zuccato C, Ciammola A, Rigamonti D, Leavitt BR, Goffredo D, MacDonald ME, et al. Loss of Huntingtin Mediated BDNF Gene Transcription in Huntington's Disease. Science. 2001;**293**(5529):493-498

[21] Bhide P, Day M, Sapp E, Schwarz C, Sheth A, Kim J, et al. Expression of Normal and Mutant Huntingtin in the Developing Brain. The Journal of Neuroscience. 1996;**16**(17):5523-5535

[22] Kalchman MA, Koide HB, McCutcheon K, Graham RK, Nichol K, Nishiyama K, et al. HIP1, a human homologue of S. cerevisiae Sla2p, interacts with membrane-associated huntingtin in the brain. Nature Genetics. 1997;**16**(1):44-53

[23] Li SH, Li XJ. Huntingtin–protein interactions and the pathogenesis of Huntington's disease. Trends in Genetics. 2004;**20**(3):146-154

[24] Harjes P, Wanker EE. The hunt for huntingtin function: interaction partners tell many different stories. Trends in Biochemical Sciences. 2003;**28**(8):425-433

[25] Ambrose CM, Duyao MP, Barnes G, Bates GP, Lin CS, Srinidhi J, et al. Structure and expression of the Huntington's disease gene: Evidence against simple inactivation due to an expanded CAG repeat. Somatic Cell and Molecular Genetics. 1994;**20**(1):27-38

[26] White JK, Auerbach W, Duyao MP, Vonsattel JP, Gusella JF, Joyner AL, et al. Huntingtin is required for neurogenesis and is not impaired by the Huntington's disease CAG expansion. Nature Genetics. 1997;**17**(4):404-410

[27] Huang EY, Zhang J, Miska EA, Guenther MG, Kouzarides T, Lazar MA. Nuclear Receptor Corepressors Partner with Class II Histone Deacetylases in a Sin3-Independent Repression Pathway. Genes & Development. 2000;**14**(1):45-54

[28] Perutz MF, Johnson T, Suzuki M, Finch JT. Glutamine repeats as polar zippers: their possible role in inherited neurodegenerative diseases. Proceedings of the National Academy of Sciences. 1994;**91**(12):5355-5358

[29] Kahlem P, Green H, Djian P. Transglutaminase Action Imitates Huntington's Disease: Selective Polymerization of Huntingtin Containing Expanded Polyglutamine. Molecular Cell. 1998;**1**(4):595-601

[30] Davies SW, Beardsall K, Turmaine M, DiFiglia M, Aronin N, Bates GP. Are neuronal intranuclear inclusions the common neuropathology of triplet-repeat disorders with polyglutamine-repeat expansions? The Lancet. 1998;**351**(9096):131-133

[31] Mitrea DM, Kriwacki RW. Phase separation in biology, functional

organization of a higher order. Cell Commun Signal. 2016;**14**:1

[32] Becher MW, Kotzuk JA, Sharp AH, Davies SW, Bates GP, Price DL, et al. Intranuclear Neuronal Inclusions in Huntington's Disease and Dentatorubral and Pallidoluysian Atrophy: Correlation between the Density of Inclusions andIT15CAG Triplet Repeat Length. Neurobiology of Disease. 1998;**4**(6):387-397

[33] Martindale D, Hackam A, Wieczorek A, Ellerby L, Wellington C, McCutcheon K, et al. Length of huntingtin and its polyglutamine tract influences localization and frequency of intracellular aggregates. Nature Genetics. 1998;**18**(2):150-154

[34] Chai Y, Koppenhafer SL, Shoesmith SJ, Perez MK, Paulson HL. Evidence for Proteasome Involvement in Polyglutamine Disease: Localization to Nuclear Inclusions in SCA3/MJD and Suppression of Polyglutamine Aggregation in vitro. Human Molecular Genetics. 1999;**8**(4):673-682

[35] Qin Z-H, Gu Z-L. Huntingtin Processing in Pathogenesis of Huntington Disease. Acta Pharmacologica Sinica. 2004;**25**(10):1243-1249

[36] Wellington CL, Ellerby LM, Hackam AS, Margolis RL, Trifiro MA, Singaraja R, et al. Caspase Cleavage of Gene Products Associated with Triplet Expansion Disorders Generates Truncated Fragments Containing the Polyglutamine Tract. Journal of Biological Chemistry. 1998;**273**(15):9158-9167

[37] Hendrick JP, Hartl FU. Molecular Chaperone Functions of Heat-Shock Proteins. Annual Review of Biochemistry. 1993;**62**(1):349-384

[38] Wyttenbach A, Carmichael J, Swartz J, Furlong RA, Narain Y, Rankin J, et al. Effects of heat shock, heat shock protein 40 (HDJ-2), and proteasome inhibition on protein aggregation in cellular models of Huntington's disease. Proceedings of the National Academy of Sciences. 2000;**97**(6):2898-2903

[39] Jana NR, Zemskov EA, Wang GH, Nukina N. Altered proteasomal function due to the expression of polyglutamine-expanded truncated N-terminal huntingtin induces apoptosis by caspase activation through mitochondrial cytochrome c release. Human Molecular Genetics. 2001;**10**(10):1049-1059

[40] Bence NF, Sampat RM, Kopito RR. Impairment of the Ubiquitin-Proteasome System by Protein Aggregation. Science. 2001;**292**(5521):1552-1555

[41] Peters MF, Nucifora FC Jr, Kushi J, Seaman HC, Cooper JK, Herring WJ, et al. Nuclear Targeting of Mutant Huntingtin Increases Toxicity. Molecular and Cellular Neuroscience. 1999;**14**(2):121-128

[42] Néri C. New light on polyglutamine neurodegenerative disorders: interference with transcription. Trends in Molecular Medicine. 2001;**7**(7):283-284

[43] Dunah AW, Jeong H, Griffin A, Kim YM, Standaert DG, Hersch SM, et al. Sp1 and TAFII130 Transcriptional Activity Disrupted in Early Huntington's Disease. Science. 2002;**296**(5576):2238-2243

[44] Sugars KL, Rubinsztein DC. Transcriptional abnormalities in Huntington disease. Trends in Genetics. 2003;**19**(5):233-238

[45] Ross CA. When more is less: Pathogenesis of glutamine repeat

neurodegenerative diseases. Neuron. 1995;**15**(3):493-496

[46] Toneff TL, Mende-Mueller Y, Wu SR, Hwang R, Bundey LM, Thompson MF, et al. Comparison of Huntingtin Proteolytic Fragments in Human Lymphoblast Cell Lines and Human Brain. J. Neurochem. 2002;**82**:84-92

Chapter 8

Brain-Derived Neurotrophic Factor and Stem Cell-Based Technologies in Huntington's Disease Therapy

Irina Kerkis, Joyce Macedo da Silva,
Cristiane Valverde Wenceslau,
Nicole Caroline Mambelli-Lisboa and Eduardo Osorio Frare

Abstract

Neurodegenerative disorders, such as Huntington's disease (HD), Alzheimer's disease (AD), and Parkinson's disease (PD), are characterized by changes in the levels and activities of neurotrophic factors (NTFs), such as brain-derived neurotrophic factor (BDNF). Gain-of-function and loss-of-function experiments demonstrate in fact the linkage between wild-type huntingtin (HTT) and gene transcription and intracellular transport of BDNF. In the present chapter, we will analyze the involvement of BDNF in HD and other neurodegenerative diseases. We will discuss the current BDNF technologies focusing on stem cell therapies that induce BDNF upregulation, for instance, the method of autologous mesenchymal stem cell (MSC) culturing in the presence of cocktail of BDNF inducers and factors (MSC/BDNF), genetic engineering of MSC and their use as a vector for BDNF gene delivery, and combined method of establishment of embryonic stem cell (ESC)-derived BDNF-overexpressing neural progenitors, which is still at the preclinical stage. Clinical trial that uses MSC/BDNF is already in course, while genetic engineering of MSC/BDNF is in perspective to treat adult and juvenile HD. The potential application of these technologies is beyond HD. Other neurodegenerative disorders such as Alzheimer's and Parkinson's diseases also can be further included in the list of clinical trials that use MSC/BDNF or even ESC/BDNF-overexpressing neural progenitors.

Keywords: brain-derived neurotrophic factor, stem cell technologies, Huntington's disease

1. Introduction

It is common knowledge that learning and memory depend on controlled signaling processes at synapses and include the precise synaptic communication between neurons and other cellular associates. Thus, the brain-derived neurotrophic factor (BDNF) and its partners appeared as key regulators of synaptic plasticity, which is the ability of synapses to increase or decrease their activity [1–3].

Generally, neuromodulators regulate neuronal plasticity; however, BDNF act as a mediator between synaptic plasticity and synaptic communication. In addition, BDNF can act in association with neurotransmitter signaling cascades showing immediate and helpful functions on synaptic plasticity [3]. Due to these properties, BDNF recently attracts much attention and became a leading strategy to stimulate neuronal and synaptic plasticity for potential protective and functionally restorative treatments for neurological and psychiatric disorders [4, 5].

Actions of BDNF in normal brain function and links between BDNF and neurodegenerative diseases suggest therapeutic potential of BDNF in diseases such as Alzheimer's disease (AD), Huntington's disease (HD), Parkinson's diseases (PD), amyotrophic lateral sclerosis (ALS), metabolic disorders (such as obesity), spinal cord injury, stroke, ischemia, etc. [6–8].

However, delivery of BDNF to the brain is challenging. The blood–brain barrier (BBB) obstructs drug delivery to the brain for the treatment of a wide range of central nervous system (CNS) diseases [9]. BDNF, a 27-kDa protein, has minimal BBB penetrability. BDNF also has a short half-life in the blood (0.92 min) and a poor pharmacokinetic profile. Systemic intravenous deliveries of BDNF are inefficient, due to the BBB, and cause strong side effects. Direct injections of BDNF into the central nervous system are invasive and limited by diffusion restrictions. Thus, alternative strategies, such as BDNF-secreting stem cells, for delivery of neuroprotective drugs are critical for promoting their clinical potentials.

2. Brain-derived neurotrophic factor

BDNF is a member of the neurotrophin family and widely expressed in the mammalian brain [1]. Precursor BDNF (proBDNF) includes an N-terminal prodomain and a C-terminal mature domain. ProBDNF is synthesized in the endoplasmic reticulum (ER) and secreted from dense-core vesicles. After packaging into dense-core vesicles, ProBDNF is trafficked through either the regulated secretory pathway or the constitutive secretory pathway [10, 11]. ProBDNF is processed to mature BDNF by several alternative cellular mechanisms. ProBDNF can be cleaved within the endoplasmic reticulum by furin or within the trans-Golgi network in regulated secretory vesicles by proconvertase enzymes. If proBDNF reaches the extracellular milieu, it can be processed by plasmin, or become endocytosed, and then cleaved to produce mature BDNF. Mature BDNF comprises dimers of the mature domain [12, 13].

BDNF can function in a highly localized manner or at a distance [14, 15]. The fact that BDNF is expressed within the peripheral ganglia and is not restricted to neuronal target fields raises the possibility that BDNF exerts paracrine or autocrine actions on neurons and non-neuronal cells [16]. BDNF binds to tyrosine receptor kinase B (TrkB) and low-affinity nerve growth factor receptor (LNGFR), also known as CD271 and p75 (NTR) [8, 17]. BDNF has been shown to modulate the activity of various neurotransmitter receptors, such as the alpha-7 nicotinic receptor [18]. BDNF has also been shown to interact with reelin, which is a large secreted extracellular matrix glycoprotein, and it supports the processes of neuronal migration and place in the developing brain through controlling cell–cell interaction signaling chain [19].

BDNF plays an important role in neurogenesis; neuronal differentiation, polarization, and guidance; and the survival of stem cells and their progenitors. The survival and differentiation of several classes of neurons in vitro, including the neural crest neurons, placode-derived sensory neurons, dopaminergic neurons in the substantia nigra, basal forebrain cholinergic neurons, hippocampal neurons,

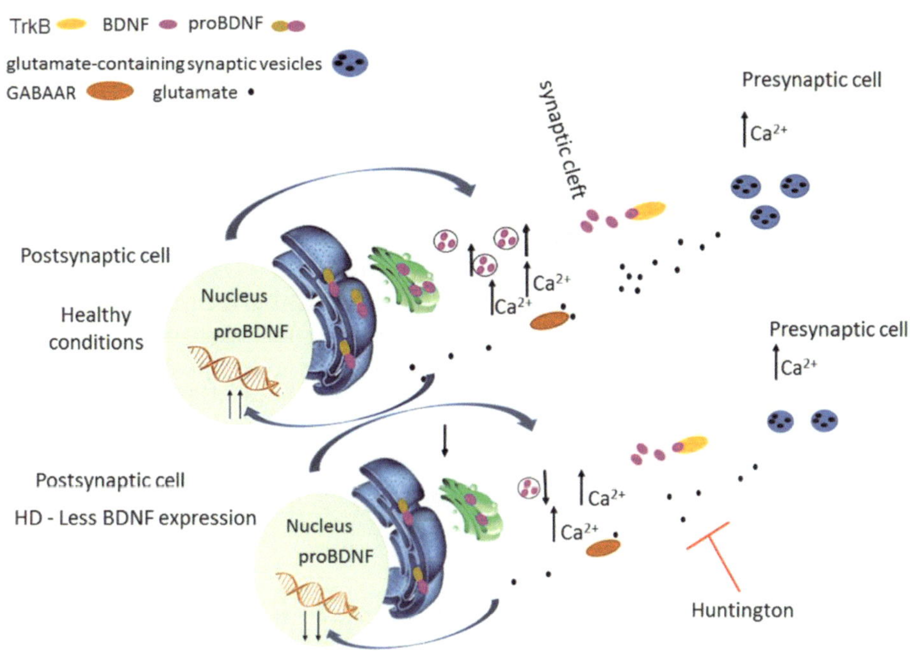

Figure 1.
The scheme of signaling involved BDNF synaptic effects and its maturation. The synthesis of BDNF from proBDNF in the endoplasmic reticulum is shown. ProBDNF binds to Golgi to enhance the proper folding of the mature domain. ProBDNF is cleaved by proteases at synapses and converted to mature BDNF. Mature BDNF binds to TrkB and glutamate released to stimulate ProBDNF transcription.

and retinal ganglia cells, are enhanced by BDNF. BDNF affects behavior by influencing the branching of differentiated neurons and the formation and maturation of spines and synapses. In the mature nervous network, amplification and enhancement of neuronal circuit structure, modulation of synaptic plasticity, and regulation of cognitive brain function (such as learning and memory) also depend on BDNF expression [4, 6–8, 20, 21].

The effects of mature BDNF are closely regulated. Even a small change in BDNF concentration may disturb the development of neural circuits and the regulation of brain function. Expression of BDNF is reduced among patients with Alzheimer's [22, 23] and Huntington's disease [7, 24]. Age-associated changes in BDNF-mediated pathways have also been shown to enhance inflammation and increase myocardial injury after myocardial infarction in the aging heart [24, 25].

The unique role of BDNF in cognitive and affective behaviors suggests their possible use to treat cognitive deficits (**Figure 1**).

3. BDNF biodistribution and serum levels in neurological and psychiatric disorders

The neocortex in the brain has morphologically stratified subdivisions into six layers: I, molecular layer; II, external granular; III, external pyramidal; IV, internal granular; V, internal pyramidal; and VI, multiform. BDNF mRNA levels vary between layers but are higher in Layer VI [26] (**Figure 2**).

The various types of afferent nerve fibers branch out in the cortex in different ways. The afferent fibers arriving from the thalamus nuclei terminate primarily in the middle layers, predominantly in the dendritic leaflets of the IV lamina.

The fibers of the other thalamic nuclei, coming from the cortical areas, ascend vertically and diffuse into different layers depending on their origin (the fibers of the thalamus intralaminal nuclei mostly terminate in Layer VI, whereas the fibers of the cortical areas terminate mainly in Layers II and III). Cortical efferent fibers, such as afferents, go to other cortical areas or to subcortical areas. Most subcortical efferences descend through the internal capsule and may or may not reach the level of the spinal cord. The blades most involved in these efferences are blade V (corticoid fibers, fibers for the brain stem and spinal cord) and lamina VI (corticothalamic fibers). Blade III is the largest source of corticocortical fibers [27].

Brain-derived neurotrophic factor is widely distributed in the central nervous system and has survival-promoting actions on a variety of CNS neurons. BDNF mRNA levels are relatively low during infancy and adolescence, peak during young adulthood, and are maintained at a constant level throughout adulthood and aging (**Figure 3**).

BDNF mRNA levels vary between layers, with Layer VI consistently higher than other layers [20, 28, 29]. The BDNF can be measured in blood samples and patients'

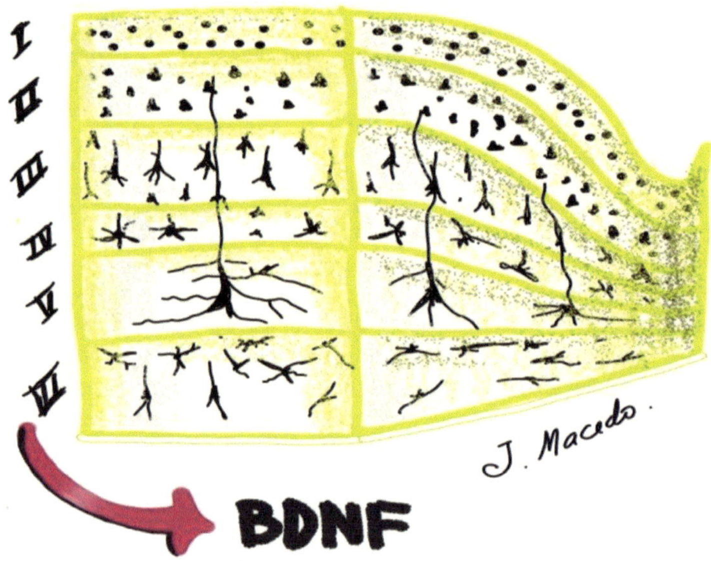

Figure 2.
Neocortex in the brain.

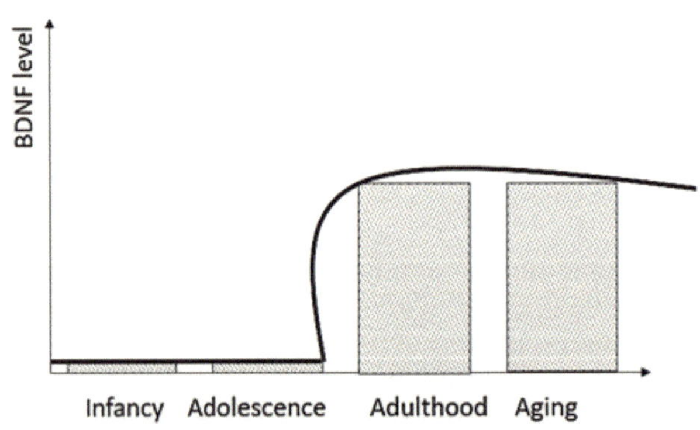

Figure 3.
BDNF throughout life.

cerebrospinal fluid. The analyses BDNF levels in CNS in neurological and psychiatric disorders showed to be different from those of normal invidious. Several studies showed a correlation between the BDNF level in serum and the clinical data for symptomatic patients [28].

Thus, the mean BDNF serum concentration was significantly lower in patients with Huntington's disease than in healthy controls ($P < 0.001$). In patients with Huntington's disease, the scale used to measure clinical parameters is Unified Huntington's Disease Rating Scale (UHDRS). The UHDRS is a clinical evaluation including domains to assess the motor, cognitive, and behavioral functions and functional capacity (Huntington Study Group, 1996).

In patients with Huntington's disease, serum BDNF levels are lower as motor and cognitive disorders progress, as measured by the UHDRS (**Figure 4**) [30].

No significant difference in BDNF levels in serum according to the subjects' gender nor significant factor modifications related to the subjects' age or to the time of day when blood was drawn ($P > 0.05$) were found [30]. A serum BDNF deficiency in HD patients is in line with the previous works highlighting trophic factor

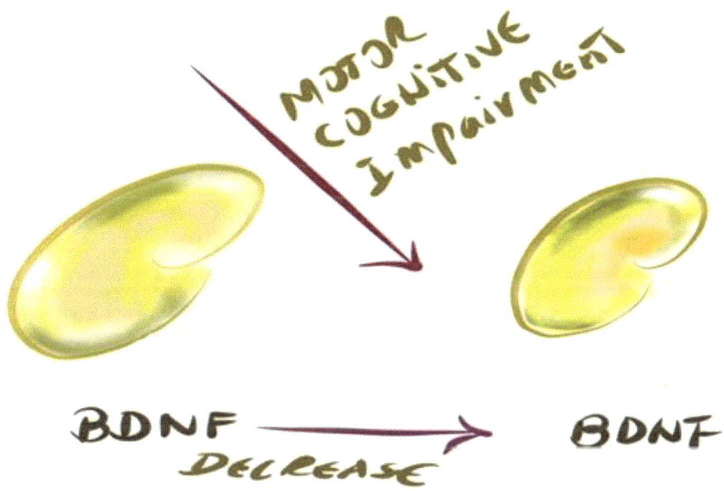

Figure 4.
BDNF decreasing with motor and cognitive impairment.

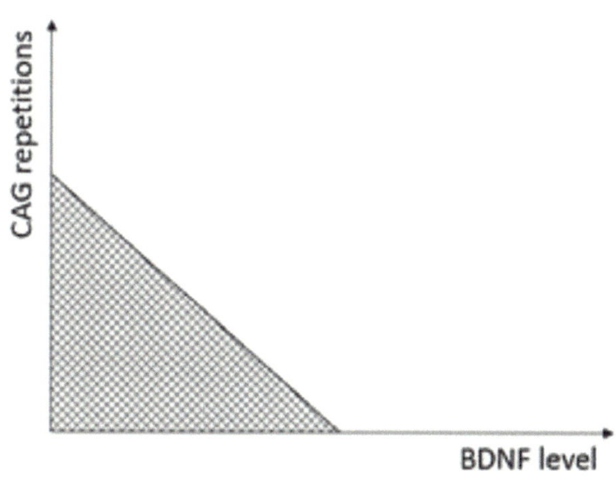

Figure 5.
Correlation between CAG repetitions and BDNF levels in patients with Huntington's disease.

dysfunction in animal models and autopsy material [31–33]. This means that BDNF levels and CAG repeats are indicators for clinical prognosis; the higher the number of CAG repeats is, the worse the prognosis, and the lower the BDNF levels are, the patient is worse clinically (**Figure 5**) [31–33].

Several lines of evidence indicate that BDNF is essential in sustaining the physiological processes of the normal, intact adult brain. BDNF has a role in modulating dendritic branching and dendritic spine morphology as well as synaptic plasticity and long-term potentiation (LTP), which is a persistent increase in synaptic strength following a high-frequency stimulation of a chemical synapse. In this manner, BDNF influences learning and memory [8, 34, 35]. BDNF also modulates hypothalamic metabolic function, further reflecting the diversity of its role in the adult brain [6].

3.1 Drugs increasing BDNF level

Some drugs may increase endogenous BDNF levels in the brain (**Figure 6**) like antidepressants, lithium, and ampakines (class of drugs that act as positive modulators of α-amino-3-hydroxy-5-methyl-4-isoxazole propionic acid (AMPA)).

These drugs are already used for symptoms that arise in diseases concomitant with neurodegenerative diseases, such as mood swings and depression. The mechanisms of action for increasing BDNF levels are still complex and not fully understood [6, 36].

3.2 Factors affecting BDNF level

Animal studies show that exercise and a calorie-restricted diet can positively affect BDNF levels in various brain regions such as the cortex and hippocampus [6]. If this pattern can be replicated in humans, this information reinforces the importance of exercise orientation and a healthy diet throughout life, especially in the young adult phase, when humans have higher levels of BDNF production in order to have good neurological performance.

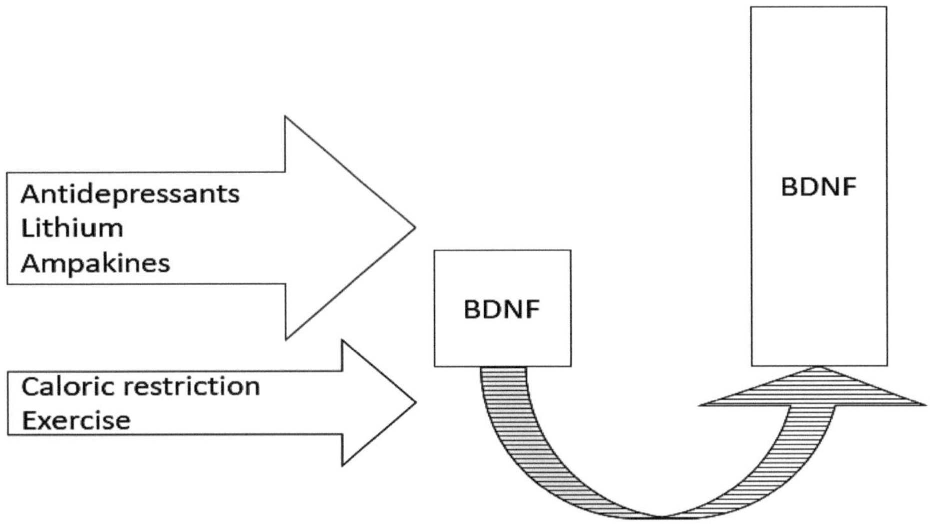

Figure 6.
Drugs and factors that increase endogenous BDNF levels.

4. BNDF therapeutic effect in neurodegenerative diseases

Neurodegenerative diseases have a continuous process of neuronal destruction and loss that can be delayed or even reversed with therapies that can improve the functional state of neurons. In theory, the earlier the diagnosis of these diseases, the greater the chance of the disease reaching a plateau and not progressing, consequently increasing the chance that the patient will preserve more functionality. Based on this therapeutic potential, growth factors have been evaluated in patients with various neurological disorders, including ALS, peripheral neuropathy, and Huntington's, Parkinson's, and Alzheimer's diseases.

4.1 Huntington's disease

Huntington's disease is a hereditary degenerative neurological disease. The most affected neurons are those that make up the extrapyramidal region but specifically the striatum (caudate and putamen nuclei). The genetic pattern of transmission is autosomal dominant, caused by the expansion of CAG triplicate repeats in the gene encoding the protein huntingtin [37].

The clinical form that expresses this lesion is evidenced by involuntary movements (chorea) in the face, trunk, and limbs, difficulty in articulating the voice, gait difficulties, and balance and cognitive decline [38–40].

In Huntington's disease, BDNF transport from the cortex to the striatum is impaired. Infusion of the BDNF protein into the striatum of HTT-mutant mice increases striatal neurons and improves motor function [39]. The use of ampakines has also been observed to increase BDNF levels in mice with beneficial results for the memory of these animals including [40].

The use of BDNF in humans would not act on the genetic cause of this disease but could slow down the progression of the disease providing a better quality of life for patients and maintaining functionality in daily activities and can be used as adjunctive therapy to currently available treatments.

4.2 Other neurodegenerative diseases

For other neurodegenerative diseases, BDNF is expected to act by improving cellular function through mechanisms involving the phosphoinositide 3-kinase and AKT and protein kinase (MEK)/extracellular signal-regulated kinase (ERK) pathway.

4.2.1 Amyotrophic lateral sclerosis

ALS is a neurological disease characterized by a progressive motor neuron atrophy, which leads to a generalized weakness and respiratory failure over a relatively rapid period of approximately 2 years. There was an old concept that ALS was an exclusively motor disease, but a cognitive impairment is now being observed as part of a frontal dementia.

The use of BDNF in this disease in both experimental animal models and later in human clinical studies could delay neuronal loss, improving the brain and spinal cord microenvironment [6].

4.2.2 Alzheimer's disease

Alzheimer's disease is a more common form of dementia and has an onset of insidious cognitive loss, progressive worsening of language, impaired visual–spatial orientation, and executive functions, and the patient has no other causes of dementia in clinical research such as infectious diseases, metabolic diseases, vascular diseases, use of medicines, and use of toxic substances, among others.

BDNF levels become deficient in the entorhinal cortex and the hippocampus in Alzheimer's disease [22, 41, 42]. A series of studies was conducted in several animal models of Alzheimer's disease to assess the effect of therapeutic application of BDNF to the entorhinal cortex [6, 43].

4.2.3 Parkinson's disease

Parkinson's disease is a neurodegenerative disorder that impairs motor function and cognitive ability. The progressive degeneration of dopaminergic neurons is reflected in the motor dysfunction of the patients.

BDNF treatment can prevent the loss of dopaminergic neurons in the substantia nigra. This is true in rodent animal models and nonhuman primates [44].

Parkinson's disease is a condition where BDNF therapy is promising and may return minimal functional and perhaps even cognitive ability to patients in the future.

5. Mesenchymal stem cell-based BDNF therapy

Mesenchymal stem cells are adult stem cells capable of self-renewal and differentiation into multiple lineages including cartilage, adipose, and bone. MSCs have been isolated from a wide range of sources including bone marrow (BM), umbilical cord, adipose tissue, multiple dental tissues, etc. Taking advantage of their multipotent, regenerative, and immunosuppressive properties, as well as tropisms to inflamed, hypoxic, and cancerous sites, MSCs have been used in various therapeutic studies, and MSC-based therapies have been shown to be safe. However, when applied alone, the efficacy in some MSC-based therapies remains low. To improve therapeutic efficacy, MSCs have been genetically modified to acquire targeted delivery function, therapeutic drug incorporation, and cell surface modification. To enhance their native properties, MSCs can also be genetically modified to overexpress therapeutic proteins.

MSCs are known to promote tissue repair by expressing a variety of bioactive molecules and secreting substances such as cytokines and growth factors. MSCs naturally secrete BDNF at low levels, varying from 0 to 200 pg/mL (**Table 1**) [45–50]. Cell therapy in regenerative medicine requires MSCs that secrete high BDNF level and are safe for use in humans.

5.1 NurOwn-MSC

BrainStorm Stem Therapeutics developed the patented NurOwn® technology that uses autologous MSCs which grow in proprietary conditions (using cocktails of inducers and factors), converting them into biological factories secreting a variety of neurotrophic factors (NTFs), including BDNF. Bahat-Stroomza et al. reported that human bone marrow-derived MSCs produced an approximately 200 pg/mL and 1400 pg/mL BDNF at baseline and after BDNF induction, respectively (**Table 1**) [46, 51]. The later was tested in humans; the bone marrow-derived MSCs did not show toxicity or side effects. Finally, Gervois et al. showed BDNF value around 2–2.5 ng/mL per $1x10^5$ MSC [52]. Currently, this technology is used in Phase 2 open-label, multicenter study of repeated intrathecal administration of autologous MSC-NTF cells in progressive multiple sclerosis. This study was designed to provide preliminary data on the safety and efficacy of these cells (**Table 2**).

5.2 MSC/BDNF and HD preclinical study

BDNF gene has been successfully introduced into MSCs using viral vectors, such as adenovirus and lentivirus (**Table 3**). Viral infections produced an 80- to 180-fold increase in BDNF production, although the absolute BDNF concentration varied significantly among the different studies (**Table 1**) [48, 53, 54] and toxicity and side effects remain unknown. More recently, preclinical double-blinded study transplanted human MSC/BDNF intrastriatal (within the corpus striatum) in two strains of immune-suppressed HD transgenic mice: YAC128 and R6/2. Following MSC/BDNF transplantation, atrophy in YAC128 mice decreased. This treatment reduced mice's anxiety that was measured in the open-field assay and increased the mean life span of the R6/2 mice. It is interesting that both MSC and MSC/BDNF transplantations induced a significant increase in neurogenesis-like activity in R6/2 mice [54]. These cells provide a platform delivery system for future studies involving corrective gene-editing strategies. Researches plan to submit an investigational new drug application to the Food and Drug Administration in order to develop Phase 1 safety and tolerability trial of MSC/BDNF in patients with Huntington's disease [55].

Cell type	Cell passage	Time of measuring (hrs)	Amount	Measure	Measure/ cell number	References
hBM-MSC	3	24	190.5	pg	5×10^5 serum free	[45]
hBM-MSC (NurOwn®)	n/if	n/if	200	pg	10^6	[46]
hBM-MSC	7–9	n/if	20–188	pg	n/if	[47]
heMSC			74–196			
hAD-MSC			35			
hBM-MSC	n/if	48	72.2	pg	—	[48]
hUC-MSC	n/if	24	50	pg	—	[49]
hWJ-MSC	n/if		37	pg	n/if	[50]

hBM-MSC, human bone marrow MSC; heMSC, human endometrial MSC; hAD-MSC, human adipose tissue-derived MSC; hUC-MSC, human umbilical cord blood MSC; hWJ-MSC, human Wharton jelly MSC; n/if, not informed.

Table 1.
BDNF secretions observed in different MSCs that naturally secrete BDNF.

Cell type	BDNF-expressing cells	Cell passage	Time of measuring (h)	Amount	Measure	Measure/ cell number	References
hBM-MSC (NurOwn®)	Wild type	n/if	n/if	200	pg	10^6	[46]
	Induced to express			1400			

Table 2.
BDNF secretions observed in BM-MSCs that naturally secrete BDNF in comparison with NurOwn BM-MSC.

Cell type	BDNF-expressing cells	Cell passage	Time of measuring (h)	Amount	Measure	Measure/ cell number	References
hBM-MSC	Adenovirus	—	48	4.73	ng	10^5	[53]
hBM-MSC	Adenovirus	—	48	643.63–13229.09 Control cells: 72.72	pg	n/if	[48]
hBM-MSC	Lentivirus	—	24	10.9–18.1	ng	2×10^5	[54]

Table 3.
BDNF secretion in BM-MSC transduced with BDNF.

6. Embryonic stem cell-derived neural progenitors/BDNF

Embryonic stem cells are pluripotent stem cells that propagated indefinitely. These cells can differentiate into cells of all three germ layers (endoderm, mesoderm, and ectoderm). ESC from teratoma and embryoid body (EB) that mimics early embryonic development. These cells differentiate efficiently into neural progenitor and functional neurons. Therefore, they can be used to differentiate into striatal medium spiny neurons (MSNs) that are lost in HD. MSNs depend on BDNF activity, and different studies try to use exogenous BDNF for striatal neuroprotection in rodent striatum HD models. Therefore, ESC and induced pluripotent stem cells (iPSC) seem to be an appropriate cell source for HD and other neurodegenerative diseases. Accordingly, ESC-derived neural progenitors overexpressing BDNF were transplanted into quinolinic acid (QA) chemical and two genetic HD mouse models (R6/2 and N171-82Q). Thus, this study combined cell replacement and BDNF supply as a potential HD therapy approach. QA-lesioned mice demonstrate the rescue of motor function by BDNF neural progenitors, while genetic mouse models showed fewer improvements. It is important to note that tumor formation was absent. The study also showed that adult neurogenesis was preserved in a BDNF-dependent manner. It was concluded that ESC-derived neural progenitors and BDNF are potential therapeutic strategies for HD to ameliorate neurodegenerative symptoms [55, 56].

7. Conclusions

It is possible to conclude that BDNF is essential for the survival, phenotypic features, and function of mature, fully developed neurons. In turn, changes in BDNF level or distribution seem to be important in the pathogenesis of neurodegenerative conditions in humans and especially in HD.

Preclinical studies over the past 20 years tested a possible neuroprotective role of BDNF in HD, which is a potent pro-survival and pro-differentiation factor for developing and adult neurons. Robust preclinical data in animals suggest that the neurotrophic action of BDNF alleviates both neuropathological and motor function deficits in the brain of patients with HD.

The intention of BDNF administration is suggested as a possible therapeutic strategy for patients with HD. However, clinical studies that used recombinant BDNF demonstrated a series of technical problems and the limited neuroprotective effects, which led to an interruption of trials with BDNF.

Based on the evidence described above, other approaches, such as stem cell-based technologies, of BDNF delivery to the brain have been developed and are currently under investigation providing promising results.

Acknowledgements

This work was supported from Cellavita Ltd., Valinhos, SP, Brazil, and Butantan Foundation, São Paulo, SP, Brazil. The funder had no role in the study design, data analysis, decision to publish, or preparation of the manuscript.

Conflict of interest

Dr. Kerkis I. received research support from Cellavita Ltd.

Author details

Irina Kerkis[1]*, Joyce Macedo da Silva[2], Cristiane Valverde Wenceslau[3], Nicole Caroline Mambelli-Lisboa[3] and Eduardo Osorio Frare[1]

1 Laboratory of Genetics, Butantan Institute, São Paulo, Brasil

2 Azidus Brasil, Valinhos, São Paulo, Brasil

3 CellAvita Ltd., Valinhos, São Paulo, Brasil

*Address all correspondence to: irina.kerkis@butantan.gov.br

References

[1] Binder DK, Scharfman HE. Brain-derived neurotrophic factor. Growth Factors. 2004;**22**:123-131. DOI: 10.1080/08977190410001723308

[2] Chao MV. Neurotrophins and their receptors: A convergence point for many signalling pathways. Nature Reviews. Neuroscience. 2003;**4**:299-309. DOI: 10.1038/nrn1078

[3] Park H, Poo MM. Neurotrophin regulation of neural circuit development and function. Nature Reviews. Neuroscience. 2013;**14**:7-23. DOI: 10.1038/nrn3379

[4] Lu B, Nagappan G, Guan X, Nathan PJ, Wren P. BDNF-based synaptic repair as a disease-modifying strategy for neurodegenerative diseases. Nature Reviews. Neuroscience. 2013;**14**:401-416. DOI: 10.1038/nrn3505

[5] Leal G, Comprido D, Duarte CB. BDNF-induced local protein synthesis and synaptic plasticity. Neuropharmacology. 2014;**76**:639-656. DOI: 10.1016/j.neuropharm.2013.04.005

[6] Nagahara AH, Tuszynski MH. Potential therapeutic uses of BDNF in neurological and psychiatric disorders. Nature Reviews. Drug Discovery. 2011;**10**:209-219. DOI: 10.1038/nrd3366

[7] Zuccato C, Cattaneo E. Brain-derived neurotrophic factor in neurodegenerative diseases. Nature Reviews. Neurology. 2009;**5**:311-322. DOI: 10.1038/nrneurol.2009.54

[8] Bathina S, Das UN. Brain-derived neurotrophic factor and its clinical implications. Archives of Medical Science. 2015;**11**:1164-1178. DOI: 10.5114/aoms.2015.56342

[9] Pardridge WM. Blood-brain barrier delivery. Drug Discovery Today. 2007;**12**:54-61. DOI: 10.1016/j.drudis.2006.10.013

[10] Aid T, Kazantseva A, Piirsoo M, Palm K, Timmusk T. Mouse and rat BDNF gene structure and expression revisited. Journal of Neuroscience Research. 2007;**85**:525-535. DOI: 10.1002/jnr.21139

[11] Al-Qudah MA, Al-Dwairi A. Mechanisms and regulation of neurotrophin synthesis and secretion. Neurosciences (Riyadh). 2016;**21**:306-313. DOI: 10.17712/nsj.2016.4.20160080

[12] Greenberg ME, Xu B, Lu B, Hempstead BL. New insights in the biology of BDNF synthesis and release: Implications in CNS function. Journal of Neuroscience. 2009;**29**:12764-12767. DOI: 10.1523/JNEUROSCI.3566-09.2009

[13] Kuczewski N, Porcher C, Lessmann V, Medina I, Gaiarsa JL. Activity-dependent dendritic release of BDNF and biological consequences. Molecular Neurobiology. 2009;**39**:37-49. DOI: 10.1007/s12035-009-8050-7

[14] Ammar MR, Thahouly T, Hanauer A, Stegner D, Nieswandt B, Vitale N. PLD1 participates in BDNF-induced signalling in cortical neurons. Science Reports. 2015;**5**:14778. DOI: 10.1038/srep14778

[15] Dechant G, Barde YA. The neurotrophin receptor p75(NTR): Novel functions and implications for diseases of the nervous system. Nature Neuroscience. 2002;**5**:1131-1136. DOI: 10.1038/nn1102-1131

[16] Gibon J, Buckley SM, Unsain N, Kaartinen V, Seguela P, Barker PA. proBDNF and p75NTR control excitability and persistent firing of cortical pyramidal neurons. The Journal of Neuroscience.

2015;**35**:9741-9753. DOI: 10.1523/JNEUROSCI.4655-14

[17] Lima Giacobbo B, Doorduin J, Klein HC, Dierckx RAJO, Bromberg E, de Vries EFJ. Brain-derived neurotrophic factor in brain disorders: Focus on Neuroinflammation. Molecular Neurobiology. 2019;**56**:3295-3312. DOI: 10.1007/s12035-018-1283-6

[18] Massey KA, Zago WM, Berg DK. BDNF up-regulates alpha7 nicotinic acetylcholine receptor levels on subpopulations of hippocampal interneurons. Molecular and Cellular Neurosciences. 2006;**33**:381-388. DOI: 10.1016/j.mcn.2006.08.011

[19] Ringstedt TA. Tale of two genes: Reelin and BDNF. In: Fatemi SH, editor. Reelin Glycoprotein: Structure, Biology and Roles in Health and Disease. New York, USA: Springer; 2008. pp. 237-238. DOI: 10.1007/978-0-387-76761-1_16

[20] Cohen-Cory S, Kidane AH, Shirkey NJ, Marshak S. Brain-derived neurotrophic factor and the development of structural neuronal connectivity. Developmental Neurobiology. 2010;**70**:271-288. DOI: 10.1002/dneu.20774

[21] Ninan I. Synaptic regulation of affective behaviors; role of BDNF. Neuropharmacology. 2014;**76**(Pt C):684-695. DOI: 10.1016/j.neuropharm.2013.04.011

[22] Ng TKS, Ho CSH, Tam WWS, Kua EH, Ho RC. Decreased serum brain-derived Neurotrophic factor (BDNF) levels in patients with Alzheimer's disease (AD): A systematic review and meta-analysis. International Journal of Molecular Sciences. 2019;**20**:257. DOI: 10.3390/ijms20020257

[23] Jiao S-S, Shen L-L, C Zhu X-LB, Liu Y-H, Liu C-H, Yao X-Q, et al. Brain-derived neurotrophic factor protects against tau-related neurodegeneration of Alzheimer's disease. Translational Psychiatry. 2016;**6**:e907. DOI: 10.1038/tp.2016.186

[24] Zuccato C, Marullo M, Vitali B, Tarditi A, Mariotti C, Valenza M, et al. Brain-derived neurotrophic factor in patients with Huntington's disease. PLoS One. 2011;**6**:e22966. DOI: 10.1371/journal.pone.0022966

[25] Kermani P, Hempstead BBDNF. Actions in the cardiovascular system: Roles in development, adulthood and response to injury. Frontiers in Physiology. 2019;**10**:455. DOI: 10.3389/fphys.2019.00455

[26] Hevner RF. Layer-specific markers as probes for neuron type identity in human neocortex and malformations of cortical development. Journal of Neuropathology and Experimental Neurology. 2007;**66**:101-109. DOI: 10.1097/nen.0b013e3180301c06

[27] Standring S. Gray's Anatomy: The Anatomical Basis of Clinical Practice. 40th ed. London, UK: Churchill Livingstone, Elsevier; 2008. p. 1584

[28] Webster MJ, Weickertb CS, Hermanb MM, Kleinmanb JE. BDNF mRNA expression during postnatal development, maturation and aging of the human prefrontal cortex. Brain Research. Developmental Brain Research. 2002;**139**:139-150. DOI: 10.1016/S0165-3806(02)00540-0

[29] Fukumitsu H, Ohtsuka M, Murai R, Nakamura H, Itoh K, Furukawa S. Brain-derived neurotrophic factor participates in determination of neuronal laminar fate in the developing mouse cerebral cortex. The Journal of Neuroscience. 2006;**26**:13218-13230. DOI: 10.1523/JNEUROSCI.4251-06.2006

[30] Ciammola A, Sassone J, Cannella M, Calza S, Poletti B, Frati L,

et al. Low brain-derived neurotrophic factor (BDNF) levels in serum of Huntington's disease patients. American Journal of Medical Genetics. Part B, Neuropsychiatric Genetics. 2007;**144b**:574-577. DOI: 10.1002/ajmg.b.30501

[31] Ferrer I, Goutan E, Marín C, Rey MJ, Ribalta T. Brain-derived neurotrophic factor in Huntington disease. Brain Research. 2000;**866**:257-261. DOI: 10.1016/s0006-8993(00)02237-x

[32] Zuccato C, Ciammola A, Rigamonti D, Leavitt BR, Goffredo D, Conti L, et al. Loss of huntingtin-mediated BDNF gene transcription in Huntington's disease. Science. 2001;**293**:493-498. DOI: 10.1126/science.1059581

[33] Baydyuk M, Xu B. BDNF signaling and survival of striatal neurons. Frontiers in Cellular Neuroscience. 2014;**8**:254. DOI: 10.3389/fncel.2014.00254

[34] Yamada K, Mizuno M, Nabeshima T. Role for brain-derived neurotrophic factor in learning and memory. Life Sciences. 2002;**70**:735-744. DOI: 10.1016/s0024-3205(01)01461-8

[35] Cunha C, Brambilla R, Thomas KL. A simple role for BDNF in learning and memory? Frontiers in Molecular Neuroscience. 2010;**3**:1. DOI: 10.3389/neuro.02.001.2010

[36] Lynch G. Glutamate-based therapeutic approaches: Ampakines. Current Opinion in Pharmacology. 2006;**6**:82-88. DOI: 10.1016/j.coph.2005.09.005

[37] Saudou F, Humbert S. The biology of Huntingtin. Neuron. 2016;**89**:910-926. DOI: 10.1016/j.neuron.2016.02.003

[38] Zuccato C, Cattaneo E. Huntington's disease. Handbook of Experimental Pharmacology. 2014;**220**:357-409. DOI: 10.1007/978-3-642-45106-5_14

[39] Bissonnette S, Vaillancourt M, Hébert SS, Drolet G, Samadi P. Striatal pre-enkephalin overexpression improves Huntington's disease symptoms in the R6/2 mouse model of Huntington's disease. PLoS One. 2013;**8**:e75099. DOI: 10.1371/journal.pone.0075099

[40] Simmons DA, Rex CS, Palmer L, Pandyarajan V, Fedulov V, Gall CM, et al. Up-regulating BDNF with an ampakine rescues synaptic plasticity and memory in Huntington's disease knockin mice. Proceedings of the National Academy of Sciences of the United States of America. 2009;**106**:4906-4911. DOI: 10.1073/pnas.0811228106

[41] Nagahara AH, Merrill DA, Coppola G, Tsukada S, Schroeder BE, Shaked GM, et al. Neuroprotective effects of brain-derived neurotrophic factor in rodent and primate models of Alzheimer's disease. Nature Medicine. 2009;**15**:331-337. DOI: 10.1038/nm.1912

[42] Giuffrida ML, Copani A, Rizzarelli E. A promising connection between BDNF and Alzheimer's disease. Aging. 2018;**10**:1791-1792. DOI: 10.18632/aging.101518

[43] Peng S, Garzon DJ, Marchese M, et al. Decreased brain-derived neurotrophic factor depends on amyloid aggregation state in transgenic mouse models of Alzheimer's disease. The Journal of Neuroscience. 2009;**29**:9321-9329. DOI: 10.1523/JNEUROSCI.4736-08.2009

[44] Mercado NM, Collier TJ, Sortwell CE, Steece-Collier K. BDNF in the aged brain: Translational implications for Parkinson's disease. Austin Neurology & Neuroscience. 2017;**2**:1021. PMID: 29726549

[45] Wilkins A, Kemp K, Ginty M, Hares K, Mallam E, Scolding N. Human

bone marrow-derived mesenchymal stem cells secrete brain-derived neurotrophic factor which promotes neuronal survival *in vitro*. Stem Cell Research. 2009;**3**:63-70. DOI: 10.1016/j.scr.2009.02.006

[46] Bahat-Stroomza M, Barhum Y, Levy YS, Karpov O, Bulvik S, Melamed E, et al. Induction of adult human bone marrow mesenchymal stromal cells into functional astrocyte-like cells: Potential for restorative treatment in Parkinson's disease. Journal of Molecular Neuroscience. 2009;**39**:199-210. DOI: 10.1007/s12031-008-9166-3

[47] Zemel'ko VI, Kozhukharova IV, Kovaleva ZV, Domnina AP, Pugovkina NA, Fridlianskaia II, et al. BDNF secretion in human mesenchymal stem cells isolated from bone marrow, endometrium and adipose tissue. Tsitologiia. 2014;**56**:204-211. PMID: 25509416

[48] Jeong CH, Kim SM, Lim JY, Ryu CH, Jun JA, Jeun SS. Mesenchymal stem cells expressing brain-derived neurotrophic factor enhance endogenous neurogenesis in an ischemic stroke model. Biomed Research International. 2014;**2014**:129145. DOI: 10.1155/2014/129145

[49] Ahn SY, Chang YS, Sung DK, Sung SI, Ahn JY, Park WS. Pivotal role of brain-derived neurotrophic factor secreted by mesenchymal stem cells in severe intraventricular hemorrhage in newborn rats. Cell Transplantation. 2017;**26**:145-156. DOI: 10.3727/096368916X692861

[50] Martins LF, Costa RO, Pedro JR, Aguiar P, Serra SC, Teixeira FG, et al. Mesenchymal stem cells secretome-induced axonal outgrowth is mediated by BDNF. Scientific Reports. 2017;7:4153. DOI: 10.1038/s41598-017-03592-1

[51] Sadan O, Shemesh N, Barzilay R, Bahat-Stromza M, Melamed E, Cohen Y, et al. Migration of neurotrophic factors secreting mesenchymal stem cells towards a quinolinic acid lesion as viewed by magnetic resonance imaging. Stem Cells. 2008;**26**:2542-2551. DOI: 10.1634/stemcells.2008-0240

[52] Gervois P, Struys T, Hilkens P, Bronckaers A, Ratajczak J, Politis C, et al. Neurogenic maturation of human dental pulp stem cells following neurosphere generation induces morphological and electrophysiological characteristics of functional neurons. Stem Cells and Development. 2015;**24**:296-311. DOI: 10.1089/scd.2014.0117

[53] Nomura T, Honmou O, Harada K, Houkin K, Hamada H, Kocsis JD. I.V. infusion of brain-derived neurotrophic factor gene-modified human mesenchymal stem cells protects against injury in a cerebral ischemia model in adult rat. Neuroscience. 2005;**136**:161-169. DOI: 10.1016/j.neuroscience.2005.06.062

[54] Pollock K, Dahlenburg H, Nelson H, Fink KD, Cary W, Hendrix K, et al. Human mesenchymal stem cells genetically engineered to overexpress brain-derived neurotrophic factor improve outcomes in Huntington's disease mouse models. Molecular Therapy. 2016;**24**:965-977. DOI: 10.1038/mt.2016.12

[55] Zimmermann T, Remmers F, Lutz B, Leschik J. ESC-derived BDNF-overexpressing neural progenitors differentially promote recovery in Huntington's disease models by enhanced striatal differentiation. Stem Cell Reports. 2016;7:693-706. DOI: 10.1016/j.stemcr.2016.08.018

[56] Reidling JC, Relaño-Ginés A, Holley SM, Ochaba J, Moore C, Fury B, et al. Human neural stem cell transplantation rescues functional deficits in R6/2 and Q140 Huntington's disease mice. Stem Cell Reports. 2018;**10**:58-72. DOI: 10.1016/j.stemcr.2017.11.005

Section 4

Amyotrophic Lateral Sclerosis: Its Genetics and Targeted Treatment Strategies

Chapter 9

Amyotrophic Lateral Sclerosis

Robin Warner

Abstract

The term motor neuron disease refers to several diseases affecting the motor neurons and is sometimes used interchangeably to refer to amyotrophic lateral sclerosis (ALS), which is the most common motor neuron disease. This chapter will focus on ALS. A complex combination of molecular pathways and cell interactions cause ALS. About 10% of ALS cases are genetic, although it has been hypothesized that as more genes are discovered to contribute to the disease, a larger percentage of cases will be quoted. This chapter discusses in detail the most common genetic forms of ALS and current research on targeted treatments.

Keywords: motor neuron disease, antisense oligonucleotide, amyotrophic lateral sclerosis, primary lateral sclerosis, novel therapies, genetics, trials

1. Amyotrophic lateral sclerosis

1.1 History of ALS

The earliest known description of motor neuron disease was in 1824 by Charles Bell, although it may have been described even earlier. The term amyotrophic lateral sclerosis was coined by Jean-Martin Charcot in his paper in 1874, where he described the condition and its connection to underlying neurological problems [1]. In 1886, Alfred Vulpian described the flail arm presentation of ALS. In 1918, Pierre Marie and his student, Patrikios, described the flail leg presentation of ALS. In 1945, the US Navy reported ALS concomitant with dementia and parkinsonism in Guam. Later, in 2011, we would know that this is due to the C9ORF72 mutation [2]. In the 1969, electrodiagnostic criteria were established for the diagnosis of ALS and updated in 2008 [3]. In 1990, the El Escorial criteria for diagnosis were established at the World Federation of Neurology meeting [4]. The first mutation related to ALS identified was the SOD1 mutation in 1993. As a result of this discovery, mouse models were created and the first medication for ALS was developed, riluzole. In 2015, the second ALS medication, edaravone, was approved [2].

1.2 Epidemiology

The most common motor neuron disease is ALS with an incidence of up to 8 per 100,000 people worldwide [5]. On average, the age of onset is 56 in sporadic ALS and 46 in familial ALS. Men are more likely to develop ALS than women. Disease duration has been quoted to be 3 years, on average; however, this is extremely variable, and it is impossible to predict the rate of decline. Cause of death is usually respiratory failure [2].

1.3 Symptoms

There are several clinical phenotypes that describe the symptom onset of amyotrophic lateral sclerosis. The classic (Charcot) phenotype is characterized by limb onset with pyramidal signs, which are not predominant [6]. This includes patients who have onset in the proximal legs. The flail arm phenotype has progressive proximal weakness and wasting in the arms for at least 12 months before the involvement of the legs or bulbar [6]. By contrast, patients with the flail leg phenotype have progressive distal onset of weakness and wasting in the legs and feet for 12 months before the involvement of the arms or bulbar. These patients are more likely to have an SOD1 mutation, with an odds ratio of 3.75 [6].

Predominantly upper motor neuron (UMN) ALS has pyramidal signs, such as severe spastic para- or tetraparesis [6]. Upper motor neuron signs, such as Babinski, Hoffmann and hyperactive reflexes or jaw jerk, are present [6]. These patients also have dysarthria or pseudobulbar affect and must show clear signs of lower motor neuron disease to differentiate them from primary lateral sclerosis [2]. This is indicated by muscle weakness or wasting, or by the presence of denervation on EMG in at least 2 different muscles [3]. These patients are more likely to have a TARDP mutation, with an odds ratio of 2.65 [6].

The bulbar phenotype has a bulbar onset of disease, characterized by dysarthria or dysphagia. They have wasting of the tongue with fasciculations on examination, and they seem to spare the limbs for at least 6 months [6]. This phenotype is more typically seen in patients with the C9ORF72 mutation with an odds ratio of 2.39 [6]. Finally, in the respiratory phenotype, prevalent respiratory impairment is apparent at onset. This may include orthopnea or dyspnea on exertion or at rest. Upper and lower motor neuron signs in this subgroup are mild in the first 6 months of disease [6].

1.4 Diagnosis

The El Escorial criteria are used to make the diagnosis of ALS [2]. They are broken down into possible, probable or definite ALS. The criteria require progression of upper and lower motor neuron deficits [4]. The signs can be clinical or electrodiagnostic (laboratory-supported ALS has been incorporated into the other categories) [3]. Definite ALS is defined by the combination of upper and lower motor neuron signs in three regions of the body, including limbs (each limb is a region) and bulbar. In probable ALS, only two regions are required, although at least one upper motor neuron sign should be more rostral. In possible ALS, only one region of both upper and lower motor neuron signs is needed. Alternatively, two regions of the upper motor neuron signs are caudal to the lower motor neuron signs [4].

Electrodiagnostic criteria of ALS have been established [3]. CMAPs should be no less than 75% of their normal value and reduction of amplitude between two points of stimulation should not be more than 30%, as this would constitute a conduction block [3]. Motor latencies and durations should be normal, or not more than 1.5 times the upper limit of normal [3]. F-response latencies should not be more than 1.3 times the upper limit of normal [3]. There should be no conduction block, as this is a sign of multifocal motor neuropathy [2]. Sensory evoked potentials should be normal in ALS [2]. On electromyography, there should be positive sharp waves, fibrillation potentials and/or fasciculation potentials in at least 2 regions [3]. Chronic neurogenic changes, such as motor unit configuration of increased duration/amplitude, polyphasia, early/reduced recruitment and increased envelope amplitude of interference pattern, are expected to be present [3].

The differential diagnosis of ALS is broad and includes infectious, inflammatory, paraneoplastic and toxic/metabolic causes [7]. Benign fasciculation syndrome is a common differential to ALS. The fasciculations in benign fasciculation syndrome are exacerbated by exercise, anxiety, caffeine, thyrotoxicosis and alcohol [7]. Only a small subset of patients who present with fasciculations progress to include other motor neuron signs. Calf fasciculations are particularly benign in nature. On electromyography, the fasciculations in ALS can double, are shorter in duration, have polyphasia and have a higher firing rate than those in benign fasciculation syndrome [4].

Multifocal motor neuropathy with conduction block has a prevalence of 0.6 per 100,000 people, which is 10 times rarer than ALS. Compared with ALS, there is a slower progression and younger onset age, and it tends to be more distal with minimal wasting [7]. Wrist drop or finger drop is a common presentation. Sensory system is not involved, unless this is a rarer form, such as MADSAM [2]. Reflexes are variable and can be brisk in up to 20% of patients. There is no bulbar or respiratory involvement [7]. The presence of conduction block on motor nerve conduction studies or triple stimulation technique (TST) is significant. Multifocal motor neuropathy and its subtypes are treatable with IVIG [2, 7].

Chronic inflammatory demyelinating polyradiculopathy has a motor predominant form that can mimic ALS [2]. The disease is symmetric with a relapsing and remitting course, which distinguishes it from ALS [7]. CSF protein elevation is important in its diagnosis and treatment is IVIG [2, 7].

Inclusion body myositis is a myopathy that mimics the anterior horn disease. Involvement of specific muscle groups, including quadriceps, wrist and finger flexors, is suspicious for this disease [2]. About 5% of these patients can have overactive reflexes and up to 40% can have fasciculations [7]. To further complicate things, electrodiagnostic studies of these patients can look more neurogenic than myogenic [7]. Quantitative motor unit analysis of the quadriceps is most sensitive in revealing a myogenic pattern with short duration units [7]. Muscle biopsy is diagnostic [2]. There is no treatment for inclusion body myositis [2].

Spinobulbar muscular atrophy is a different motor neuron disease caused by an x-linked polyglutamine mutation with CAG repeats in the androgen receptor gene [2]. This makes the androgen receptor less functional and causes atrophy and weakness in bulbar and limb girdle muscles [2]. Endocrine signs, such as gynecomastia, diabetes mellitus and testicular atrophy, differentiate this from ALS [7]. There is no treatment for spinobulbar muscular atrophy [2, 7].

Primary progressive multiple sclerosis can mimic ALS; however, this is easily excluded with MRIs of the neuroaxis or the presence of oligoclonal bands in the CSF [7]. Myasthenia gravis, particularly MUSK, may mimic ALS [7]. Myasthenia gravis is characterized by fatigable weakness, differentiating it from the weakness of ALS [2]. Serum antibody testing can differentiate myasthenia gravis from ALS [7].

Infectious causes of motor neuron mimic syndromes include human T-lymphotropic virus (HTLV) and West Nile virus, as well as post-poliomyelitis syndrome [7]. Polio infections affect the anterior horn cells [2]. West Nile virus has an associated myelitis, among other neurologic symptoms [2]. HTLV causes a demyelinating upper motor neuron disease called tropical spastic paraparesis [7]. Bladder dysfunction and sensory changes differentiate this from ALS [7].

1.5 Current treatments

The mainstay of treatment at this time is riluzole [2]. Edaravone is also approved for the treatment of ALS; however, its intravenous administration and requirement of a port leads to complications [8]. An oral form of Edaravone is being developed.

A third approved drug, a combination of dextromethorphan and quinidine, has been beneficial for pseudobulbar affect and other bulbar dysfunction in ALS [2].

Respiratory function is monitored using forced vital capacity (FVC) every 3 months [9]. It is more accurately done lying down [9]. Unfortunately, FVC is not a good measure of early respiratory decline and can be confounded by the inability to create an adequate seal on the mouthpiece [9]. Respiratory failure in ALS is best treated with the use of noninvasive ventilation (NIV) [2]. These methods include cough assist early on and then may advance to BiPAP [9]. Invasive ventilation, such as intubation and tracheostomy, are options for emergent respiratory support or severe respiratory failure in ALS; however, there will be a difficult decision to withdraw invasive respiratory support, should the patient worsen. Early discussion of advanced directives (before dementia or inability to communicate) is essential to prevent unwanted invasive procedures in an emergency [9].

Physical and occupational therapy can help improve function by training patients in compensatory skills and providing assistive devices for every step of the way. A study that looked at exercise in ALS showed there is no risk of worsening disease with moderate exercise [10]. Low-impact aerobic exercises can improve cardiovascular health and decrease depressive symptoms [10]. Speech-language pathology is important for tracking bulbar dysfunction and giving advice on how to speak more clearly or modify foods and drink to prevent choking [10].

Maintaining weight using a high-calorie diet has been shown to improve quality of life and survival in patients with ALS [11]. More studies on which macronutrients are most beneficial are needed, although current studies show that high-fat and high-cholesterol diets are beneficial [11]. If bulbar dysfunction progresses to the point where the patient cannot eat or drink without choking, or if the patient loses more than 5% of his or her body weight between visits (3 months), a feeding tube (usually a percutaneous endoscopic gastrostomy, or PEG) is recommended [11]. Unfortunately, there is weak evidence that PEG tubes prolong survival, despite benefits of reducing weight loss, preventing dehydration and administration of medications [11].

The future of directed treatments for ALS is bright. Later in this chapter, I will discuss research into the treatment of genetic ALS.

2. Genetic amyotrophic lateral sclerosis

About 10% of ALS cases are genetic [2]. Most are autosomal dominant, although they can be recessive or X-linked [2]. Over 30 genes related to ALS have been discovered so far. The most common of these are C9ORF72 (about 30% in Europeans and 2.3% in Asians), SOD1 (14.8% in Europeans and 30% in Asians), TAR DNA-binding protein (4.2% in Europeans and 1.5% in Asians) and fused in sarcoma (2.8% in Europeans and 6.4% in Asians) [12]. Ubiquilin2 (UBQLN2), ALSIN, senataxin (SETX), spatacsin, vesicle-associated membrane protein-associated protein B (VAPB), angiogenin (ANG), factor-induced gene 4 (FIG 4), optineurin (OPTN) and "other unknown genes" account for the rest [2]. Only a few of these, such as C9ORF72, are causal. The rest are disease-modifying genes [12].

2.1 C9ORF72 and SETX

C9ORF72 is a protein differentially expressed in normal and neoplastic cells, which modulate (via Rab or Ras GTPase) endosomal trafficking and autophagy in primary neurons [12, 13]. The gene is located on chromosome 9p21.2 and is a hexanucleotide repeat of GGGGCC [2]. In a healthy person, there are 20–30 repeats;

however, someone with the mutation can have hundreds of repeats [13]. Although anticipation is shown in trinucleotide repeat disorders, it has not been demonstrated in hexanucleotide repeat disorders [14]. Repeats are typically expanded in multiples of 3 to preserve the genetic reading frame [15]. Most repeat disorders do not cause catastrophic frame shift mutations, unless a stop codon is the triplet added [15]. There is a transitional number between the normal number of repeats to the permutation and finally to the number of repeats that determine a mutation, although exact numbers are currently not agreed upon in ALS [13].

Typically, after inheritance of a repeat expansion, it remains dormant in the cell [13]. As the cells divide, the repeats tend to continue to expand when more repeats are copied onto the daughter strands during replication [13]. Repeat DNA is more susceptible to damage [15]. Fibroblasts and lymphocytes from patients with Huntington's disease, ALS, Alzheimer's disease and Parkinson's disease all have DNA that is relatively sensitive to ionizing radiation and chemical mutagens [15]. When the damaged DNA is repaired, more repeats are created during DNA repair [15]. Mismatch and base-excision repair cause somatic expansion of repeated sequences of trinucleotide repeat disorders [15]. As this in more cells, the organism eventually reaches a critical point at which a significant number of cells meet the threshold number of repeats to produce disease [13, 15]. Progression of disease occurs when more cells reach this threshold and enter a pathologic state [13, 15].

Repeat expansion mutations in the C9ORF72 gene, such as the hexanucleotide repeat seen in ALS, lead to the formation of R-loops in the DNA [16]. R-loops are a hybridization of mRNA with dsDNA with looped intron sequences, which have been spliced out of the mRNA during the transcription process [16]. R-loops occur naturally in several cellular processes, including mitochondrial DNA replication, and in the transcription bubble [16]. R-loops have been thought to rarely occur as transcriptional by-products but are more common than once thought [16]. Others believe that R-loops are natural intermediates of transcription that are eliminated by Senataxin [17].

RNA:DNA hybrids are more stable than dsDNA [16]. High G-content (like in the C9ORF72 hexanucleotide repeat) encourages and stabilizes R loops by facilitating the opening of the transcriptional bubble while DNA strands are still separated [16]. SETX is one of the genes involved in terminating transcription and senataxin depletion (such as in SETX ALS) correlates with the accumulation of RNA:DNA hybrids [17]. The mRNA would usually move out of the nucleus and not interact with the dsDNA as much; however, this mRNA becomes sequestered in the nucleus [16]. This enlarges the nucleolus and recruits the cell DNA damage response [16]. If unsuccessful, the DNA damage response will signal for apoptosis of the neuron [16].

Haploinsufficient proteins form from translated GGGGCC introns that are not degraded after splicing [18]. These are exported out of the nucleus by an unknown mechanism and translated in the cytoplasm [18]. The resulting haploinsufficient C9ORF72 protein forms toxic dipeptide aggregates that accumulate in the neuron [18]. These haploinsufficient proteins may have properties of prions [18].

2.2 SOD

SOD (superoxide dismutase) is a cytoplasmic enzyme of 153 amino acids: one copper atom for function and one zinc atom for structural stability [18]. It converts oxygen radicals into peroxide and oxygen [18]. The cell is then able to turn the peroxide into water and oxygen with catalase [18]. This is an extremely stable protein, but can unfold from dimer to two unfolded monomers via a folded monomer intermediate step [18]. A complex combination of molecular pathways and cell interactions cause ALS [2]. Oxidative stress, aberrant RNA processing and protein misfolding/insoluble proteins have all been implicated in motor neuron degeneration in ALS [2]. This is an example of an oversimplified mechanism of SOD1-mediated ALS. Microglia secrete cytokines, stimulating inflammation by recruiting astrocytes [18]. Astrocytes come and release nitric oxide and prostaglandin E2 [18]. SOD comes to convert NO into peroxide and oxygen [18]. In ALS patients, the SOD that arrives is mutated and aggregates, leading to endoplasmic reticulum (ER) stress [18]. The ER helps with endosomal trafficking, so defective endosomal trafficking causes organelle disruption, including mitochondrial disruption, and activates apoptosis of the neuron [18]. ER stress also causes dysfunction in axonal transport, leading to axonal loss [18].

The SOD1 gene is located on chromosome 21q22 [2] and contains 5 exons [18]. About 150 mutations of this gene have been identified, which are predominantly missense mutations, but also include nonsense mutations, insertions and deletions [2]. Notable mutations in this group include SOD1A4V-ALS for its rapid clinical progression, SOD1A89V-ALS for its sensory neuropathy, SODI113T-ALS for its diversity of phenotype and SOD1G93A-ALS for its use in transgenic mice [2, 18]. The SOD1D90 mutation is recessive in Scandinavians, but dominant in other groups [18]. SOD1 knockout mice do not develop clinical ALS [18]. Instead, they develop age-dependent distal motor neuropathy, suggesting a toxic gain of function in the SOD [18].

2.3 FUS and TAR DNA-binding protein

FUS is a DNA- and RNA-binding protein that repairs damage and breaks, especially double-strand breaks in DNA [19, 20]. Loss of function mutations in FUS gene (16p11.2) lead to impairment of the poly(ADP-ribose) polymerase (PARP)-dependent DNA damage response, leading to increased DNA damage, especially in neurons [19]. The mutated FUS aggregates [19]. In ALS, the mutations are located in the nuclear localization sequence in the c-terminus [19]. This causes FUS to lose its ability to stay in the nucleus and the mutated FUS will instead aggregate in the cytoplasm [19]. ALS due to the TARDBP gene has a similar mechanism also with cytoplasmic aggregates [20]. Inclusion bodies that are FUS positive, TDP-43 negative may be found [19]. The typical phenotype for FUS-ALS is a lower motor neuron predominant syndrome without bulbar involvement [2]. They may have frontotemporal dementia as well [2]. The typical age at onset ranges from as young as the mid-twenties to as late as the eighth decade of life [2]. Mean duration of this form of ALS is 33 months [2].

3. Genetic treatments

3.1 CRISPR

CRISPR (clustered regularly interspaced short palindromic repeats) was discovered in 1987 in Osaka by Ishino et al. in *E. coli*, although their significance was unknown [21]. The CRISPR/Cas system is a part of the prokaryotic immune system, allowing resistance to foreign genetic data from bacteriophages [21]. Archaea and bacteria use CRISPR/Cas to find bacteriophage DNA that has been entered into its genome and remove it [21].

There are three steps of CRISPR/Cas-mediated immunity [21]. The first step is adaptation [21]. Prokaryotes place protospacers in their DNA made up of pieces of foreign DNA (from phages and plasmids that previously invaded) attached to palindromic repeats [21]. The second step is expression with maturation [21]. Transcription of the protospacers and repeats yields a precursor CRISPR-RNA, which will mature into the guide RNA (gRNA) [21]. The third step is interference [21]. Once mature, the guide RNA is used in the CRISPR/Cas system to recognize and create a double-strand break by foreign DNA [21].

Pieces of foreign DNA are stored by the prokaryote in the form of a genetic library of phages and plasmids, which have previously invaded [21]. Cas (CRISPR-associated protein) scans bacterial DNA for bacteriophage DNA that matches the guide RNA attached to CRISPR and cleaves it, when found [21]. Cas is a DNA endonuclease that allows for unwinding of DNA, checking for sites complementary to the guide RNA (20 BP spacer region) [21]. Once a match is found, it cleaves both strands of the DNA [21]. When the cell attempts to repair the break, mutations are often introduced, deactivating the viral gene [21]. The repair can be done via nonhomologous end joining (NHEJ), which can be done at any point in the cell cycle. In certain stages of the cell cycle, homology-directed repair (HDR) occurs, allowing for more precise DNA repair [21]. Researchers have been working on enhancing this type of repair for high-fidelity CRISPR/Cas-mediated gene editing [22]. This process can be manipulated for gene inactivation or insertion of foreign DNA [22]. Mammalian cells predominantly rely on nonhomologous end joining for DNA repair, which is error-prone, resulting in insertion and deletion (indels) mutations [21]. Specifically in neurons, which are terminally differentiated post-mitotic cells, homology-directed repair is limited, but nonhomologous end joining is easier [22].

3.2 Use of CRISPR in eukaryotes

In 2012, Jennifer Doudna from UC Berkeley and Emmanuelle Charpentier from Umea University in Sweden demonstrated the use of CRISPR/Cas for human controlled genetic editing [21]. She fused CRISPR RNA (crRNA) with trans-activating CRISPR RNA (tacrRNA) to form a chimeric single-guide RNA (sgRNA) to allow for site-specific gene editing in a eukaryote [21]. This method is popular due to its low cost and ease of production in a lab [21]. Since then, research in CRISPR has expanded to include every species: from attempts to drive malaria-carrying mosquito species to extinction to combating antibiotic resistance to agriculture, making crops hardier [21].

Unfortunately, the CRISPR/Cas9 system is not specific enough to prevent it from cleaving nontarget DNA [21]. DNA does not have to fully match the guide RNA (can tolerate 3–5 mismatches) for it to introduce a double-strand break, which leads to unpredictable mutations [21]. Researchers have been working to increase the specificity of CRISPR/Cas9 systems by using two guide RNAs or shorter (truncated) guide RNAs [22]. Decreasing the GC content of guide RNAs also helps specificity [23]. Adding a short-lived ribonucleoprotein to the CRISPR-Cas9 system decreases off-target effects by allowing the complex to break down after a short period of activity [22]. This allows for more locally acting gene editing. There is also the possibility of introducing the Cas protein instead of the Cas gene into a subject, so the effect on the genome is shorter-lived [22].

There are other downsides, including immune attacks on the system, due to its bacterial origin [21]. PEGylation, the modification of biomolecules by adding polyethylene glycol (PEG), a nontoxic, nonimmunogenic polymer, is one method to circumvent immune attack [21]. Humanization of the proteins is another method of circumventing this problem [22].

3.3 Cas modification and types

The Cas protein may be modified in many different ways, including deactivating one or both cutting domains and adding deaminases, transcriptional activators or blockers (dCas-sgRNA) [22]. Deactivating one of the cutting domains, creating a 'nick' instead of a 'break,' prevents unwanted damage in off-target sites [22]. One may opt to deactivate both cutting domains (dead Cas or dCas) and attach other enzymes to the complex, such as deaminases, which cause point mutations [22]. These point mutations may include stop codons to prevent transcription of a disease gene (CRISPR interference CRISPRi), or they may change a disease-causing mutation to a healthy gene [23]. Transcriptional activators, such as VP64 or MS2 coat protein, may be added to recruit transcription machinery and promote transcription of specific genes (CRISPR activation or CRISPRa) [21]. CRISPRi is accomplished by adding a Kruppel-associated box (KRAB) domains to inactivate transcription by recruiting factors that physically block the gene [21].

Alternatively, one can use a different type of Cas. Each bacterial species has its own Cas protein, or multiple types of Cas [22]. Strep. pyogenes Cas9 (spCas9) was found first and is most commonly used in a CRISPR type II system, may be directed by two guide RNAs [22]. Cas9 cuts double-stranded DNA that matches the guide RNA [21]. Staph. aureus Cas9 (saCas9) is small, which allows it to fit inside adeno-associated virus, making it a convenient choice for that vector [24]. Strep. thermophilus Cas9 (stCas9) is more specific, requiring a match to not only the guide RNA but also a protospacer-adjacent motif (PAM) (a specific sequence next to the viral DNA) [24]. This prevents unwanted off-target effects. CasX is the smallest known Cas so far and less immunogenic [25]. Jennifer Doudna discovered CasX, found in ground-dwelling bacteria, which are unfamiliar to the human immune system and nonpathologic, decreasing the chance of immunogenicity [25]. Cas12 cuts double-stranded DNA that matches the guide, as well as all single-stranded DNA in a cell in a nonspecific way [21]. Cas13 cuts all single-stranded RNA in a cell [21]. Cas14 is found in Archaea and is very small [22]. It cuts all single-stranded DNA in a cell in a more specific way, with a system (DETECTR) that detects infectious organisms and genetic mutations [22]. Cpf1 is an endonuclease that leaves an overhang on one side of the double-strand break (DSB), which promotes nonhomologous end joining in neurons [21].

Delivery methods for the CRISPR/Cas system include viral vectors, nanoparticles, lipofectamine, nucleofection, microinjection, short-lived ribonucleoproteins and electroportation [23]. Some of these methods, including microinjection and electroportation, can damage cells and are not possible in vivo [23]. In electroportation, an electric field increases permeability of cell membrane, allowing entry of the CRISPR/Cas system into the cell [23]. Nucleofection, nanoparticles and lipofectamine are less commonly used by researchers due to the tendency for low cell penetrance using these methods [23]. Viral vectors are the most common and effective delivery systems. AAV (adeno-associated viral vector) is the most commonly studied vector [26, 27]. The limiting factors in the use of viral vectors are low cargo capacity, immunogenicity and tissue specificity [26]. AAV is a small virus that does not cause disease, just a very mild immune response [26]. It attaches and infiltrates the host cell. The virus transfers DNA into the nucleus, leading to sustained gene expression [26]. There is ~ 4.7 kb AAV vector packaging limit [26]. Therefore, when using this delivery system with spCas9, two AAVs are required: one to package spCas9 and the other to package the sgRNAs [26]. With smaller Cas types, such as saCas9, only one AAV is required [26]. AAV is specific to muscle, liver, brain and eye tissue [27]. Immune response (mainly humoral, due to prior infection with AAV) was found in 96% of patients in one study [27]. These patients demonstrated antibodies for AAV [26, 27]. Other delivery systems use other viruses, such as adenovirus and lentivirus [26]. Short-lived ribonucleoproteins (RNP) are proteins that shuttle the CRISPR-Cas system into a cell [27]. Since they are short-lived, the action of the CRISPR-Cas system tends to be local to where the RNPs are injected [27]. These decrease off-target effects and are less immunogenic than viral vectors [23].

3.4 Antisense oligonucleotides

Antisense oligonucleotides (ASOs) are synthetic nucleic acid sequences that bind RNA to modulate gene expression [28]. ASOs can restore protein function by splice modification, decrease aberrant protein function by silencing, modify protein function or reduce toxicity of an aberrant protein [28]. ASOs penetrate their target with the help of ribose alteration, avoid degradation by nucleases and avoid immune response by alterations in their phosphate group, ribose and nucleosides [28]. Two ASOs were FDA approved in 2016: eteplirsen for Duchenne muscular dystrophy and nusinersen for spinal muscular atrophy [28]. Proteinuria has been a common side effect with the ASOs, although it has been mostly benign [28].

About 14% of patients who have Duchenne muscular dystrophy contain the mutation at exon 51, where eteplirsen takes action [29]. It works by mRNA knock-down via activation of RNA-H, which breaks down the RNA-DNA complex before translation [29]. It aims to skip the mutated exon to convert the frame shift mutation back into the reading frame [29].

Nusinersen works via alteration of gene splice site [30]. It targets intronic splicing silencer N1 (ISSN1), causing inclusion of exon 7 in SMN2 pre-mRNA [30]. This results in SMN2 protein translation that looks identical to SMN1 protein [30].

CRISPR-Cas systems have some benefit over ASOs, such as being less cytotoxic and requiring less number of treatments [23].

3.5 Other methods of genetic manipulation

Meganucleases are large endonucleases, able to cut out large, 14–40 base pair (BP) long, DNA sequences [31]. They were discovered in the 1980s [31]. Although these are specific, they are costly to create, requiring expertise and more time than CRISPR, which makes it inefficient [31]. Meganucleases have been studied in Duchenne muscular dystrophy [31]. One group designed a meganuclease that cuts upstream of the deletion ‘hot spot’ of intron 44 of the dystrophin gene [31]. It was delivered via a lentiviral vector [31]. After administration, expression of a fully corrected dystrophin gene was observed via western blot [31].

Zinc finger nucleases recognize short sequences (3 BP) of DNA, but can be combined with several other zinc fingers to accommodate longer sequences [32]. They are less specific, but are expensive to make as they require expertise, time and effort to create [32]. They are cytotoxic to cells, so currently, they are mainly in use for modifying stem cells and immune cells [32]. Ousterout et al. used this technology in myoblast cell cultures to yield dystrophin expression [32].

Transcription activator-like effector nuclease (TALEN) are artificial restriction enzymes, fused to a nuclease and designed to recognize specific DNA sequences of 33 or 34 amino acid repeats [33]. They are able to perform DNA repair, replacement, insertion or deletion [33]. This is a precise method that is easy to make and is not costly [33]. TALEN has been used successfully in human cell cultures (myoblasts and dermal fibroblasts) with Duchenne muscular dystrophy, as well as to treat Golden Retrievers with muscular dystrophy [33].

RNA interference (RNAi) is used in the cell to control gene expression [34]. Two types of RNAs are known to perform this function: small interfering RNAs (siRNA) and microRNAs (miRNA) [34]. After RNA polymerase II produces mRNA, the mRNA travels to the cytoplasm for transcription, unless it is intercepted by RNA interference [34]. siRNA or miRNA binds to enzymes that break down mRNAs that match or closely match a sequence in them [34]. miRNAs are about 21 nucleotides long and bind to dicer, an enzyme that cleaves mRNA that matches the single-stranded microRNA [34]. After cleavage, the mRNA is degraded [34]. Argonaut is another enzyme that performs the same function [34]. Once bound to miRNA or siRNA, the complex is called RISC (RNA-induced silencing complex) [34]. siRNAs differ from miRNAs in that they are double stranded [34]. RNAi requires multiple treatments and can be cytotoxic [34].

4. Use of genetic treatments in treating motor neuron disease

4.1 CRISPR treatment of ALS

Treatment of ALS has been limited by the limited understanding of the mechanism of disease [2]. Some of the use of CRISPR/Cas9 research done in ALS is to identify the mechanism by which the various genes cause toxicity, discovering modifiers and RNA-processing pathways [35].

Researchers did a proof of concept study, which demonstrated that using CRISPR/Cas9 in an AAV delivery system in G93A-SOD1 mice targeting the SOD1 mutation has delayed onset, increased survivability of motor neurons, decreased motor atrophy, increased motor function and prolonged lifespan, compared to control mice [36]. G93A-SOD1 transgenic mice were infused at birth or first day of life with the delivery system [36]. Typically, the mice develop symptoms at 90 days of life [36]. A single peptide is changed in the SOD1 mutation in this model [36]. The amount of mutant SOD1 protein in the spinal cord was reduced by the infusion, compared with control mice [36]. This delayed the onset of disease by a range of 2–36 days, but did not slow disease progression once the onset came [36]. However, the delay in onset prolonged survival in test mice by 25%, compared to diseased controls [36].

Another group was able to produce gene-corrected fibroblast stem cells using a CRISPR/Cas9 system from ALS patients with SOD1 and FUS mutations [37]. They first collected and cultured FUS and SOD1-mutated fibroblasts and confirmed their mutations [37]. Then, they used a CRISPR/Cas system with electroportation to target the FUS mutation for correction with single-stranded oligodeoxynucleotide as a repair template [37].

In 2017, researchers demonstrated that they could use genetically modified mesenchymal stem cells to express neurotrophic factors [38]. Neurotrophic factors are peptides that promote growth, survival and differentiation of neurons [38]. This paper proposes that CRISPR/Cas in an AAV delivery system is a good way to genetically modify mesenchymal stem cells to express these factors, which are neuroprotective [38].

Other researchers are looking at using CRISPR/Cas13 to target aberrant mRNAs in C9ORF72 ALS patients [39]. CRISPR/Cas13 cuts RNA and this group modified it to be more specific toward the toxic mRNAs, which do not leave the nucleus and lead to R-loops in DNA [39]. Their mouse models have shown improvement in motor symptoms [39].

This group [40] was able to eliminate toxic microsatellite repeat expansion RNAs with an RNA-targeting Cas9 in myotonic dystrophy cell cultures. They developed a programmable CRISPR/Cas9 system to visualize and eliminate repetitive RNAs retained and aggregating in the nucleus [40]. Although these experiments were conducted in myotonic dystrophy cell cultures, not cell cultures expressing C9ORF72, they are theoretically applicable [40].

In 2018, a group did a genome-wide survey, looking for suppressors and enhancers of C9ORF72 dipeptide repeat toxicity in human cells [41]. These were validated using primary mouse neurons with CRISPR/Cas9 screening [41]. They discovered several modifiers, but one in particular, called TMX2, modulated the endoplasmic reticular stress caused by C9ORF72 dipeptide repeats, increasing survival to 100% (from 10%) in their mouse models [41].

Additional researchers used a SaCas9 endonuclease to disrupt HERV-K env, a retroviral gene, human mouse mammary tumor virus-like 2, related to prostate cancer motor neuron disease [42]. They found this inhibited molecules involved in amyotrophic lateral sclerosis, including epidermal growth factor receptor (EGF-R), nuclear factor kappa-light-chain-enhancer of activated B cells (NF-κB), SF2/ASF and TDP-43 [42]. These molecules are important for RNA-binding and alternative splicing [42].

4.2 ASO editing of ALS

Tofersen is an antisense oligonucleotide that binds to the mRNA from the SOD1 gene [43]. This drug is being studied in patients with ALS caused by the SOD1 mutation [43]. In the phase 1/2 trial, treatment with tofersen 100 mg in 10 patients with SOD1 fALS over a three-month period resulted in a statistically significant lowering of SOD1 protein levels in the cerebrospinal fluid and a slowed decline in the ALS Functional Rating Scale-Revised (ALSFRS-R) compared to 12 patients receiving a placebo [44]. They also noted slowed decline in muscle strength and vital capacity in the study group [44].

5. Conclusion

Amyotrophic lateral sclerosis is a disease with no cure; however, current research is promising for a cure in the near future. Technologies in genetic editing show particular promise in the field of neurodegeneration. Molecular mechanisms of genetic diseases, even those with known mechanisms, are oftentimes much more complex than initially thought. Discoveries regarding transcription modulators have proven particularly useful in research to find treatments for ALS. Given the recent advances in these areas, the future appears brighter for patients with ALS.

Acknowledgements

I would like to thank the Muscular Dystrophy Association for their support.

I would like to acknowledge Dr. Dale Lange for inspiring my interest in neuromuscular medicine.

My program director, Dr. Dora Leung, was instrumental in defining the path of my career. For this, I am extremely grateful.

Conflict of interest

The author declares no conflict of interest.

Author details

Robin Warner
Department of Neurology, Hospital for Special Surgery, New York, NY, USA

*Address all correspondence to: warnerr@hss.edu

References

[1] Goetz CG. Amyotrophic lateral sclerosis: Early contributions of Jean-Martin Charcot. Muscle & Nerve. 2000;**23**:336-343. DOI: 10.1002/(SICI)1097-4598(200003)23:3<336::AID-MUS4>3.0.CO;2-L

[2] Anthony A, James R. Neuromuscular disorders. In: Chapter 6: Amyotrophic Lateral Sclerosis. 2nd ed. 2015. pp. 174-193

[3] Carvalho M et al. Electrodiagnostic criteria for diagnosis of ALS. Clinical Neurophysiology. 2008;**119**:497-503. DOI: 10.1016/j.clinph.2007.09.143

[4] Ludolph A, Drory V, Hardiman O, Nakano I, Ravits J, Robberecht W, et al. A revision of the El Escorial criteria. Amyotrophic Lateral Sclerosis and Frontotemporal Degeneration. 2015;**16**(5-6):291-292. DOI: 10.3109/21678421.2015.1049183

[5] Longinetti E, Fang F. Epidemiology of amyotrophic lateral sclerosis: An update of recent literature. Current Opinion in Neurology. 2019;**32**(5):771-776. DOI: 10.1097/WCO.0000000000000730

[6] Chiò A, Moglia C, Canosa A, Manera U, D'Ovidio F, Vasta R, et al. ALS phenotype is influenced by age, sex, and genetics: A population-based study. Neurology. 2020;**94**(8):e802-e810. DOI: 10.1212/WNL.0000000000008869

[7] Ghasemi M. Amyotrophic lateral sclerosis mimic syndromes. Iranian Journal of Neurology. 2016;**15**(2):85-91

[8] Yoshino H. Edaravone for the treatment of amyotrophic lateral sclerosis. Expert Review of Neurotherapeutics. 2019;**19**(3):185-193. DOI: 10.1080/14737175.2019.1581610

[9] Pirola A, De Mattia E, Lizio A, Sannicolò G, Carraro E, Rao F, et al. The prognostic value of spirometric tests in amyotrophic lateral sclerosis patients. Clinical Neurology and Neurosurgery. 2019;**184**:105456

[10] Lewis M. The role of physical therapy and occupational therapy in the treatment of amyotrophic lateral sclerosis. NeuroRehabilitation. 2007;**22**(6):451-461. DOI: 10.3233/NRE-2007-22608

[11] Ludolph AC, Dorst J, Dreyhaupt J, Weishaupt JH, Kassubek J, Weiland U, et al. Effect of high-caloric nutrition on survival in amyotrophic lateral sclerosis. Annals of Neurology. 2020;**87**:206-216. DOI: 10.1002/ana.25661

[12] Mathis S, Goizet C, Soulages A, Vallat JM, Masson GL. Genetics of amyotrophic lateral sclerosis: A review. Journal of the Neurological Sciences. 2019;**399**:217-226. DOI: 10.1016/j.jns.2019.02.030

[13] Van Mossevelde S, van der Zee J, Gijselinck I, et al. Clinical evidence of disease anticipation in families segregating a C9orf72 repeat expansion. JAMA Neurology. 2017;**74**(4):445-452. DOI: 10.1001/jamaneurol.2016.4847

[14] Shin JW, Kim K-H, Chao MJ, Atwal RS, Gillis T, MacDonald ME, et al. Permanent inactivation of Huntington's disease mutation by personalized allele-specific CRISPR/Cas9. Human Molecular Genetics. 2016;**25**(20):4566-4576. DOI: 10.1093/hmg/ddw286

[15] Massey TH, Jones L. The central role of DNA damage and repair in CAG repeat diseases. Disease Models & Mechanisms. 2018;**11**:dmm031930. DOI: 10.1242/dmm.031930

[16] Wahba L, Koshland D. The Rs of biology: R-loops and the regulation

of regulators. Molecular Cell. 2013;**50**(5):611-612. DOI: 10.1016/j.molcel.2013.05.024

[17] Mischo Hannah E, Gómez-González B, Grzechnik P, Rondón AG, Wei W, Steinmetz L, et al. Yeast Sen1 helicase protects the genome from transcription-associated instability. Molecular Cell. 2011;**41**(1):21-32. DOI: 10.1016/j.molcel.2010.12.007

[18] Andersen PM. Amyotrophic lateral sclerosis associated with mutations in the CuZn superoxide dismutase gene. Current Neurology and Neuroscience Reports. 2006;**6**:37-46. DOI: 10.1007/s11910-996-0008-9

[19] Nauman M, Pal A, Goswami A, Lojewski X, Japtok J, Vehlow A, et al. Impaired DNA damage response signaling by FUS-NLS mutations leads to neurodegeneration and FUS aggregate formation. Nature Communications. 2018;**9**:335. DOI: 10.1038/s41467-017-02299-1

[20] Chou C, Zhang Y, Umoh ME, et al. TDP-43 pathology disrupts nuclear pore complexes and nucleocytoplasmic transport in ALS/FTD. Nature Neuroscience. 2018;**21**:228-239. DOI: 10.1038/s41593-017-0047-3

[21] Simpson BP, Davidson BL. Nervous system drug delivery. Chapter 18: CRISPR-Cas Gene Editing for Neurological Disease. London, UK: Academic Press; 2019. pp. 365-376. DOI: 10.1016/B978-0-12-813997-4.00018-9

[22] Raschmanová H, Weninger A, Glieder A, Kovar K, Vogl T. Implementing CRISPR-Cas technologies in conventional and non-conventional yeasts: Current state and future prospects. Biotechnology Advances. 2018;**36**(3):641-665. DOI: 10.1016/j.biotechadv.2018.01.006

[23] Kruminis-Kaszkiel E, Juranek J, Maksymowicz W, Wojtkiewicz J. CRISPR/Cas9 technology as an emerging tool for targeting amyotrophic lateral sclerosis (ALS). International Journal of Molecular Sciences. 2018;**19**(3):906. DOI: 10.3390/ijms19030906

[24] Steinert J, Schmidt C, Puchta H. Use of the Cas9 Orthologs from Streptococcus thermophilus and *Staphylococcus aureus* for non-homologous end-joining mediated site-specific mutagenesis in *Arabidopsis thaliana*. In: Schmidt A, editor. Plant Germline Development. Methods in Molecular Biology. Vol. 1669. New York, NY: Humana Press; 2017

[25] Liu J, Orlova N, Oakes BL, et al. CasX enzymes comprise a distinct family of RNA-guided genome editors. Nature. 2019;**566**:218-223. DOI: 10.1038/s41586-019-0908-x

[26] Daya S, Berns KI. Gene therapy using adeno-associated virus vectors. Clinical Microbiology Reviews. 2008;**21**(4):583-593. DOI: 10.1128/CMR.00008-08

[27] Gregorevic P, Blankinship M, Allen J, et al. Systemic delivery of genes to striated muscles using adeno-associated viral vectors. Nature Medicine. 2004;**10**:828-834. DOI: 10.1038/nm1085

[28] Goyal N, Narayanaswami P. Making sense of antisense oligonucleotides: A narrative review. Muscle & Nerve. 2018;**57**:356-370. DOI: 10.1002/mus.26001

[29] Nathalie G et al. A randomized placebo-controlled phase 3 trial of an antisense oligonucleotide, drisapersen, in Duchenne muscular dystrophy. Neuromuscular Disorders. 2018;**28**(1): 4-15. DOI: 10.1016/j.nmd.2017.10.004

[30] Finkel RS, Chiriboga CA, Vajsar J, Day JW, Montes J, De Vivo DC, et al. Treatment of infantile-onset

spinal muscular atrophy with nusinersen: A phase 2, open-label, dose-escalation study. Lancet. 2016;**388**(10063):3017-3026. DOI: 10.1016/S0140-6736(16)31408-8

[31] Popplewell L, Koo T, Kymäläinen H, Leclerc X, Duclert A, Mouly V, et al. Meganuclease-enhanced genome correction therapy for Duchenne muscular dystrophy. Neuromuscular Disorders. 2012;**22**:S9. DOI: 10.1016/S0960-8966(12)70015-9

[32] Ousterout DG, Kabadi AM, Thakore PI, Perez-Pinera P, Brown MT, Majoros WH, et al. Correction of dystrophin expression in cells from Duchenne muscular dystrophy patients through genomic excision of exon 51 by zinc finger nucleases. Molecular Therapy. 2015;**23**(3):523-532. DOI: 10.1038/mt.2014.234

[33] Mata López S, Balog-Alvarez C, Vitha S, Bettis AK, Canessa EH, Kornegay JN, et al. Challenges associated with homologous directed repair using CRISPR-Cas9 and TALEN to edit the DMD genetic mutation in canine Duchenne muscular dystrophy. PLoS One. 2020;**15**(1):e0228072. DOI: 10.1371/journal.pone.0228072

[34] Hannon G. RNA interference. Nature. 2002;**418**:244-251. DOI: 10.1038/418244a

[35] Chan D, Chan G, Palczewski K, Lewis K, Ho J. CRISPR for treating ALS - A long and bumpy road ahead. Rare Disease Reviews. 2019. DOI: 10.13140/RG.2.2.12995.25120

[36] Gaj T, Ojala DS, Ekman FK, Byrne LC, Limsirichai P, Schaffer DV. In vivo genome editing improves motor function and extends survival in a mouse model of ALS. Science Advances. 2017;**3**(12):eaar3952. DOI: 10.1126/sciadv.aar3952

[37] Wang L, Yi F, Fu L, Yang J, Wang S, Wang Z, et al. CRISPR/Cas9-mediated targeted gene correction in amyotrophic lateral sclerosis patient iPSCs. Protein & Cell. 2017;**8**(5):365-378. DOI: 10.1007/s13238-017-0397-3

[38] Zhang Z, Zhang Y, Gao F, Han S, Cheah KS, Tse HF, et al. CRISPR/Cas9 genome-editing system in human stem cells: Current status and future prospects. Molecular Therapy--Nucleic Acids. 2017;**9**:230-241. DOI: 10.1016/j.omtn.2017.09.009

[39] Smargon AA, Shi YJ, Yeo GW. RNA-targeting CRISPR systems from metagenomic discovery to transcriptomic engineering. Nature Cell Biology. 2020;**22**:143-150. DOI: 10.1038/s41556-019-0454-7

[40] Nelles D, Pirie E, Blue S, Marina R, Wang H, Chaim I, et al. Elimination of toxic microsatellite repeat expansion RNA by RNA-targeting Cas9. Cell. 2017;**170**(5):899-912.e10. DOI: 10.1016/j.cell.2017.07.010

[41] Kramer NJ, Haney MS, Morgens DW, Jovičić A, Couthouis J, Li A, et al. CRISPR/Cas9 screens in human cells and primary neurons identify modifiers of C9ORF72 dipeptide-repeat-protein toxicity. Nature Genetics. 2018;**50**(4):603-612. DOI: 10.1038/s41588-018-0070-7

[42] Ibba G, Piu C, Uleri E, Serra C, Dolei A. Disruption by SaCas9 endonuclease of HERV-Kenv, a retroviral gene with oncogenic and neuropathogenic potential, inhibits molecules involved in cancer and amyotrophic lateral sclerosis. Viruses. 2018;**10**:412. DOI: 10.3390/v10080412

[43] Cappella M, Ciotti C, Cohen-Tannoudji M, Biferi MG. Gene therapy for ALS—A perspective. International Journal of Molecular Sciences. 2019;**20**:4388. DOI: 10.3390/ijms20184388

[44] Abati E, Bresolin N, Comi G, Corti S. Silence superoxide dismutase 1 (SOD1): A promising therapeutic target for amyotrophic lateral sclerosis (ALS). Expert Opinion on Therapeutic Targets. 2020;**24**(4):295-310. DOI: 10.1080/14728222.2020.1738390

Section 5

Prions in Health and Disease

Chapter 10

Electrophysiological Investigations of Prion Protein Roles in Health and Disease

Simote T. Foliaki, Bradley R. Groveman and Cathryn L. Haigh

Abstract

Prion diseases are transmissible and fatal neurological disorders associated with the misfolding of cellular prion protein (PrPC) into disease-causing isoforms (PrPD) in the central nervous system. The diseases have three etiologies; acquired through exposure to the infectious PrPD, sporadic, arising from no known cause, and hereditary due to familial mutations within the *PRNP* gene. The manifestation of clinical signs is associated with the disruption of neuronal activity and subsequent degeneration of neurons. To generate insight into the mechanisms by which neuronal activity becomes disrupted in prion diseases, electrophysiological techniques have been applied to closely study the electrical signaling properties of neurons that lack functional PrPC as well as neurons that are developing pathological features of prion diseases due to infection or genetic mutation. In this review, we will compile the electrophysiological evidences of neurophysiological roles of PrPC, how those roles are changed in neurons that are developing prion diseases, and how disease-associated effects are exacerbated during the clinical stage of disease.

Keywords: prion, CJD, LTP, electrophysiology, PrPC roles

1. Introduction

Prion diseases are transmissible neurological disorders that are always fatal following symptom onset. These diseases affect humans and animals. The most common forms in humans are Creutzfeldt-Jakob disease (CJD), Gerstmann-Straussler-Scheinker syndrome (GSS), and familial fatal insomnia (FFI). The primary causative event is the misfolding of PrPC into PrPD in the central nervous system, which is followed by progressive impairments of cognition and behaviour. The fundamental roots of the clinical manifestations are the impairments of neuronal activity. In patients, these changes are mostly detected by electroencephalography (EEG) and functional magnetic resonance imaging (fMRI) [1]. The abnormal neuronal activities associated with prion diseases have been successfully modeled in the laboratory using mouse models, cultured mouse primary neurons, and cultured human/mouse induced pluripotent stem cells [2, 3]. As a result of advancements in experimental neuro-electrophysiology technologies, our understanding of neuroelectrical signaling dysfunctions associated with prion diseases has substantially improved over the last decades.

IntechOpen

In experimental models, there have been several neuro-electrophysiological phenomena identified in the glutamatergic neuronal system that closely correlate with the underlying molecular mechanisms of memory formation/loss and behavioral change. These include the short-term plasticity (STP), long-term potentiation (LTP), and long-term depression (LTD) [4]. STP is usually detected as a rapid physiological alteration of neuronal activity that lasts milliseconds to seconds immediately after neurons receiving a stimulation [5, 6]. This short-term function is usually due to a rapid enhanced release of neurotransmitters that overwhelmingly activate the preexisting receptors on the post-synaptic terminals [5, 6]. Through such a mechanism, STP can be evoked by a paired-stimulus delivered a few milliseconds apart, in which the post-synaptic response evoked by the second stimulus indicates the probability of neurotransmitter release at a synapse or a population of synapses [5, 6]. Further, with repetitive short (~0.5–1 min) trains of high frequency (~100–200 Hz) stimulation, neurotransmitters are released at a substantial level, which extensively depolarizes the post-synaptic membrane causing activation of the NMDA receptor (NMDAR), a glutamate receptor that modulates the post-synaptic currents when it is active [7]. The post-synaptic response within seconds of the high frequency stimulation is largely STP, reflecting the levels of neurotransmitters release [8]. Repetitive stimuli can also evoke a short-term phenomenon called the afterhyperpolarization, which usually lasts 1 second. Afterhyperpolarization is divided into three parts, the fast (first few milliseconds), medium (100–500 milliseconds), and slow (longer than 500 milliseconds) afterhyperpolarization [9]. The afterhyperpolarization is largely dependent on the activity of potassium channels, especially the calcium-sensitive potassium channels, as well as the activity of voltage-gated calcium channels and the level of intracellular calcium [9, 10].

The activation of NMDARs following a repetitive high frequency stimulation causes externalization of more AMPA receptors (AMPARs). AMPARs are a type of glutamate receptor known as the workhorse of glutamatergic neurons because they can rapidly generate synaptic signaling [7]. The rapid recruitment of AMPARs can subsequently activate neighboring silent synapses, causing excitatory neurons to remain persistently active for hours, a phenomenon called LTP [11]. On the other hand, repetitive and prolonged (~5–10 min) trains of low frequency (~0.5–5 Hz) stimulation cause depolarization of post-synaptic membrane and activation of NMDARs in a way that triggers internalization of AMPARs, causing depression of the post-synaptic current that can persist for hours, a neuro-phenomenon called LTD [4]. While these are the main known mechanisms of LTP and LTD, the fast-growing interest on how these phenomena are induced and maintained has led to the discovery of a wide variety of potential molecular mechanisms.

To understand the mechanisms underlying the neuronal dysfunctions associated with the clinical phenotypes of prion diseases, studies have focused on identifying how the neuro-electrophysiological correlates of cognition and behaviour become impaired in experimental models of disease. In this review, we will discuss the normal neuro-electrophysiological roles of PrPC and the neuro-physiological alterations during the asymptomatic stage to the early onset of clinical signs in models of acquired and genetic prion diseases.

2. Neuro-electrophysiology of PrPC

PrPC is a membrane-tethered glycoprotein, targeted to the outer leaflet of the plasma-membrane by a glycosylphosphadiylinositol (GPI) anchor. The precise functions of PrPC in the central nervous system are largely unknown; however,

Roles of PrPC in cell functions and signaling	Reference
Neurotransmitter release	[13, 18–20]
Long-term potentiation	[22–24]
Metaplasticity	[27]
Calcium-dependent potassium channel function	[20, 22, 30]
L-type voltage-gated potassium channel function	[10, 20]
NMDA receptor function	[14]
Voltage-gated calcium channel function	[36]
Calcium homeostasis	[10, 20]
GABA receptor function	[14, 22, 30, 38]
Maintenance of peripheral nerves myelination	[40]
Modulator of various signaling functions including Fyn and mGluR5 dependent regulation of NMDAR activity, and modulation of p38 Mitogen Activated Protein Kinase signaling pathway (refer to the subheading: *PrPC regulates major intracellular signaling pathways*)	[33, 42]

Table 1.
Summary of the normal physiological roles of PrPC including the studies that reported those roles.

there is considerable evidence to suggest that PrPC has important roles in neuronal activity [12] (**Table 1**). These putative functions of PrPC have been studied by combinations of electrophysiological recordings, genetic modifications, and pharmacological approaches.

2.1 PrPC assists synaptic transmission

PrPC is expressed in both pre- and postsynaptic terminals [13–19], where it plays essential roles in synaptic activity. PrPC interacts with presynaptic vesicles and facilitates release of neurotransmitters [13, 20, 21]. PrPC also regulates presynaptic calcium channels, allowing influx of sufficient calcium into the presynaptic terminal to facilitate the release of neurotransmitters [21, 22]. At the post-synaptic terminals, PrPC interacts with various post-synaptic glutamate receptors and regulates their functions (discussed later in this section) [14, 23]. In mice devoid of PrPC expression, it has been found that LTP within the hippocampal CA1 and dentate gyrus is significantly impaired [24–26]. This impairment is associated with memory and behavioral deficits [27]. However, this is still a point of contention as normal LTP within these regions has also been observed and the discrepancy appears un-related to the genetic background of the mouse model [5, 28–30]. Hippocampal CA1 metaplasticity is also impaired in PrP knockout mice; here the post-synaptic responses become enhanced as opposed to being depressed when a low frequency stimulation is paired with a couple trains of theta-burst stimulation (consists of 10 trains delivered at 5 Hz where each train comprises of 4 pulses delivered at 100 Hz) at an interval of ~25 minutes [29]. Further, Juvenile PrP knockout mice exhibit poor sensorimotor performance, which correlates with the cerebellar granule cells displaying slow rate of inward and outward membrane currents, slow kinetics of excitatory post-synaptic responses, and incompetence to induce LTP by theta-bust stimulation [31]. These abnormal phenotypes disappear when the mice reach adulthood [30, 31], thus suggesting that PrPC plays some essential roles in synaptic transmission during early development.

2.2 GPI-anchored PrPC regulates ion channels activity

The activity of ion channels is essential for the maintenance of synaptic functions [7]. The involvement of PrPC in ion channel activity has been implicated in mice lacking PrPC [12]. These mice exhibit electrophysiological features of dysfunctional ion channels such as reduced slow and medium afterhyperpolarization in the hippocampal CA1 region, which indicates an impairment of calcium-dependent K^+ channels [22, 24, 32]. This finding is consistent with the report that PrPC modulates the activity of voltage-dependent potassium channels [33]. Additionally, the hippocampal CA1 exhibits reduced currents of L-type voltage-gated calcium channels in the absence of PrPC [22], albeit another study showed the contradictory finding [10]. In cultured hippocampal neurons from PrP knockout mice, the activity of NMDARs is significantly impaired. These receptors exhibit a longer decay time and larger amplitude of miniature synaptic currents as well as very slow deactivation kinetics of agonist-mediated currents [14]. The interpretation of these findings was that PrPC functions to prevent hyperactivation of NMDARs.

The contribution of PrPC to ion channel activity has also been reported in a variety of cells expressing PrPC with various primary sequence mutations; designed to determine the effect of each mutant on ion channel activity as a measure of prion neurotoxicity [34]. Several deletions (between residues 94 and 134) in the charged and hydrophobic region of PrP, a conserved region of PrP, cause dysfunction of cation-permeable channels, which increases the inward currents leading to cellular toxicity and cell death [34–36]. The deletion of PrP residues 105–125 or 94–134 causes the most deleterious dysfunction of ion channels. Deletion of other residues such as PrP 94–110, 111–134, and 114–121 also causes similar toxic effect, but at relatively lower degrees [35]. Although these observations have mostly been reported in nonneuronal cells (HEK293T) [34–36], the neonatal death in mice expressing PrP devoid of 105–125 residues affirms that the deleterious effect of this deletion appears independent of cell type [37].

When PrP residues 105–125 are co-deleted with residues 51–90 (a five octapeptide repeat region), the impairment of ion channels becomes slightly reduced [35]. Furthermore, the toxic effect of PrP lacking residues 105–125 vanishes when co-deleted with either the GPI anchor (PrP 231–254) alone or the GPI anchor and the endogenous signal motif (PrP 1–22; to retain PrP in the cytoplasm), suggesting that the toxic PrP needs to be transported out of the cytoplasm and anchored to the lipids in order to disrupt the activity of ion channels. This evidence implies that GPI-anchored PrPC prevents hyperactivity of ion channels. Further support for this role has also been observed using cells lacking GPI-anchored PrP, where the calcium current intensity of voltage-gated calcium channels (containing subunits $Ca_V2.1/\beta$ and $\alpha2\delta$-1 or $\alpha2\delta$-2) becomes reduced in the presence of GPI-anchored PrP but enhanced in the presence of only GPI-anchorless PrP [38]. Taken together, when PrPC is correctly trafficked and anchored to the cell membrane, it regulates the activity of ion channels, predominantly through its charged and hydrophobic region.

2.3 PrPC maintains neuronal calcium homeostasis

As aforementioned, PrPC regulates ion channels including the voltage-gated calcium channels and NMDARs. In the absence of endogenous PrPC expression, hippocampal CA1 neurons exhibit dysfunction of calcium homeostasis associated with diminished currents of Nifedipine-sensitive voltage-gated L-type calcium-channels [22]. This finding contradicts another showing that voltage-gated calcium channels are not affected in PrP knockout hippocampal neurons despite exhibiting impaired slow afterhyperpolarization, suggesting that the disruption of calcium homeostasis is less likely to be due to a dysfunction or loss of voltage-gated calcium channels [10]. In a study by Powell et al., they revealed that the calcium uptake into the ER, a calcium storage mechanism essential for normal cellular calcium homeostasis, was abnormally enhanced in PrP knockout neurons [10]. This dysfunction, together with the reduced amplitude of slow afterhyperpolarization, was significantly rescued following pharmacological inhibition of the sarcoplasmic/ER pump calcium-ATPase [10]. Together, these data suggest that PrPC regulates intracellular calcium homeostasis largely by controlling ER calcium uptake, which subsequently alters the activity of voltage gated calcium channels.

2.4 PrPC regulates function of inhibitory neurons

Mice devoid of PrPC expression exhibit weak GABA(A) receptor-mediated fast inhibition in the hippocampal CA1 region [24]. The inhibiting role of GABAergic neurons in the glutamatergic transmission is important to ensure no hyperactivity of the excitatory neurons [39]. This weak GABAergic neuronal activity in the absence of PrPC is consistent with other reports of enhanced excitability in the hippocampal CA1 and dentate gyrus of PrP knockout mice [14, 32, 40]. Importantly, the hyperactivity of excitatory neurons together with the weak function of GABA(A) receptor agrees with the report that PrP knockout mice are susceptible to kainite-induced epileptic seizure [40]. However, a study of the olfactory bulb in PrPC lacking mice has shown an enhanced inhibitory postsynaptic currents are received by mitral cells, which appears associated with the depressed high-frequency oscillations during a single breath [41]. Altogether, PrPC appears to differentially regulate inhibitory neuronal activity based on location; where in the hippocampus it enhances the inhibitory activity to prevent excitotoxic death, the olfactory bulb it prevents hyperactivity of the inhibitory cells to maintain normal high frequency oscillations [41].

2.5 PrPC maintains myelination of nerve cells

One of the abnormalities detected in mice lacking PrPC expression is the demyelination of peripheral nerve cells [42]. The loss of PrPC in neurons, but not in Schwann cells, triggers chronic demyelination, which causes significant reduction in peripheral nerve conduction velocity [42]. This dysfunction can be prevented by re-introduction of PrPC expression as well as by activation of PrPC proteolysis [42], thus indicates that PrPC is necessary for maintaining the integrity of myelin sheath. This finding helps consolidating locomotion deficits such as reduced capability to explore an open field, nest, swim, and groom, which have been reported in aged PrP knockout mice [27, 43]. However, it is not yet known whether PrPC also displays this function in the central nervous system.

2.6 PrPC regulates major intracellular signaling pathways

PrPC anchoring to the cell membrane is thought to be essential for its role in signaling functions [35, 44]. Several downstream signaling pathways of PrPC have been identified following the discovery of its role as a receptor in neurotoxicity of amyloid beta and alpha-synuclein oligomers [15, 45]. These oligomers bind to PrP residues 95–105 [46] and mediate activation of the signaling intermediate Fyn tyrosine kinase by mGluR5, which causes overactivation of NMDARs leading to excitotoxicity and cell death [15, 45]. Similarly, NMDAR is also overactivated by infectious and toxic PrPD species binding to membrane PrPC, likely through the same mechanistic pathway as the oligomers of amyloid beta and alpha-synuclein, which subsequently activates the p38 Mitogen Activated Protein Kinase signaling pathway and induces neurotoxicity [23]. The activation of these downstream signaling pathways significantly disrupts both the propagation of action potentials and synaptic functions leading to impairment of LTP and LTD [15, 23, 45, 47, 48]. Together, the evidence suggests that, indirectly, PrPC normally acts as an upstream modulator of a wide variety of intracellular signaling pathways that are essential for neuronal activity.

3. Neuro-physiology during prion diseases

Because the underlying mechanisms by which neuronal functions become impaired following the misfolding of PrPC to PrPD and the accumulation of PrPD remain largely unknown, studies have been focused on determining how the roles of PrPC in neuronal activity become altered during disease. However, these mechanisms may be influenced by how PrPC gets misfolded into PrPD. There are three etiologies of prion disease; exposure to infectious prions (acquired), familial disease-related mutations within *prnp*, or undergoing unknown cellular events that cause sporadic prion disease. To date, there has been no way to identify cells that might develop sporadic prion disease due to its unknown cause. However, the causes of acquired and genetic prion diseases can be identified, allowing these diseases to be modeled in the laboratory. These models of prion diseases have provided significant insights to physiological changes in cells prior to clinical onsets.

During the clinical stage of either acquired or genetic prion diseases, significant degeneration of neurons has occurred, as well as the pathological features specific to prion diseases such as spongiosis, deposition of PrPD including the protease-resistant species, and production of potent self-propagating PrPD [49–51]. The degeneration of neurons impedes studies attempting to further understand pathogenic mechanisms during this stage of the disease for two main reasons. Firstly, the degeneration of neurons is almost solely responsible for all neuronal dysfunctions at the clinical stage [51, 52]. Second, neuronal degeneration is irreversible; attempts to rescue mice that have already undergone neuronal degeneration only prolong the disease progression in the terminal stages to death [53]. In addition, recent studies have reported that at the clinical stage of CJD, the peripheral nerves are also severely demyelinated (**Figure 1(6)**) [54, 55], supporting that therapeutic drug interventions at this stage might be too late. Hence, studies have shifted interests toward understanding changes during the preclinical stage to early onset of clinical signs at which points the neurodegeneration is very minimal and therapeutic interventions have been successful in mice [56]. Since electrophysiological paradigms can detect neuronal dysfunctions during the asymptomatic stage as well as the early symptomatic stage, studies have utilized these paradigms to further understand molecular mechanisms that may lead to therapeutic development against neuronal degeneration.

3.1 Acquired prion diseases

When mice expressing endogenous PrPC are exposed to infectious PrPD, they will develop prion disease, usually over a well-defined (strain-specific) period of time [57, 58]. Hence, it is possible to study biochemical and physiological properties of mouse neuronal cells during the asymptomatic stage prior to the onset of clinical disease. The hippocampal CA1 LTP is significantly impaired in wild type mice infected with mouse-adapted scrapie (ME7) before the onset of clinical

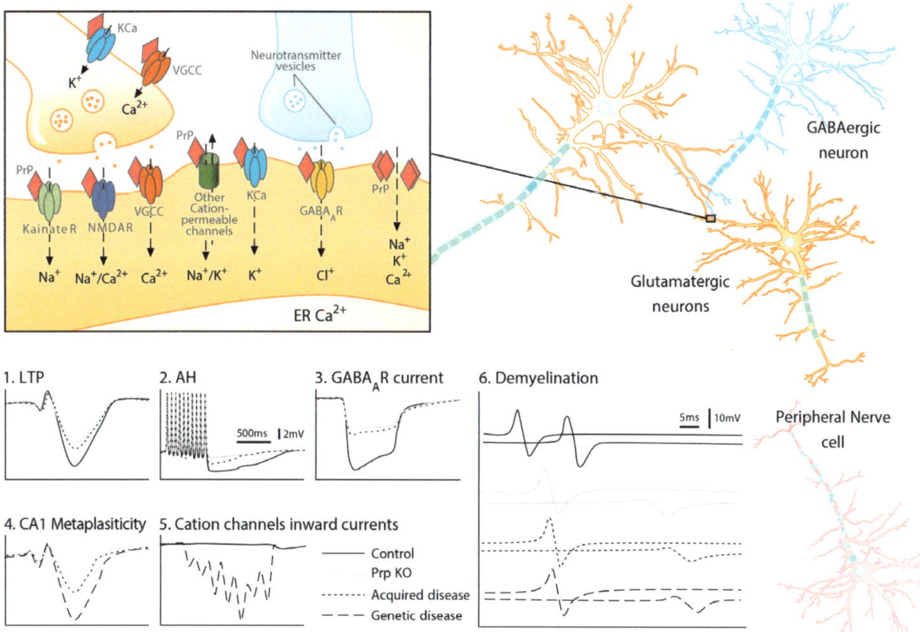

Figure 1.

Connections between the neuro-physiological changes during diseases pathogenesis and the loss or corruption of PrPC function. The neurons in the low magnification (top right side) are CNS neurons with normal myelin sheath. These neurons include two glutamatergic neurons (yellow) and one GABAergic neurons (blue) that form dendrodendritic synapses (as visualized in high magnification). The neuron at the bottom right corner is a peripheral nerve cell with demyelination. Relative to wild type mice expressing PrPC without the disease: 1—hippocampal LTP is impaired in mice lacking PrPC as well as in mice developing prion disease caused by infection; 2—the amplitudes of medium and slow afterhyperpolarizations (AHs) are reduced in PrP knockout (KO) mice and wild type mice during the early symptomatic stage of prion disease caused by exposure to infectious PrPD; 3—GABA(A) receptor currents are weak in PrP knockout mice as well as in disease caused by PrPD infection; 4—hippocampal CA1 metaplasiticity is abnormally enhanced in mice harboring the D178N/129V mutation and slightly enhanced in PrP knockout mice; 5—inward ion currents through cation-permeable channels are abnormally increased in cells expressing P101L, G113V, and G130V; 6—peripheral nerve cells are demyelinated in both PrP knockout mice as well as in disease. 1–5—These dysfunctions are likely due to changes in activities of several key receptors/ion channels, known to interact with PrP, in excitatory (Glutamatergic) and inhibitory (GABAergic) neurons.

signs (**Figure 1(1)**) [51, 59]. This impairment of LTP strongly correlates with the increased levels of synaptic PrPD [59]. A similar finding has been reported in hamsters infected with hamster-adapted scrapie PrPD (Sc237) [60]. The LTP dysfunction indicates an overall synaptic transmission abnormality (**Figure 1**). Because PrP regulates activities of various receptors in both pre- and postsynaptic terminals that are essential for the induction and maintenance of LTP, the disruption of LTP is likely a result of the functions of these receptors being altered during disease. From as early as 30 days post inoculation (dpi) in the neocortex layer five and 50 dpi in the hippocampal CA1, before the early onset of clinical disease (70–80 dpi), the medium and late afterhyperpolarizations become significantly impaired (**Figure 1(2)**) [60]. This finding suggests a significant calcium dysregulation at this stage of the disease, which is believed to be due to a significant disruption of certain voltage-gated calcium channels such as those activated by potassium or from a significant failure of intracellular calcium storage systems to store or release calcium [60]. In addition, the activity of GABA(A) receptor is hindered in GPI−/− mice infected with scrapie during the early stage of the disease (**Figure 1(3)**) [61]. This finding appears consistent with the reports of the close interaction between GABA(A) receptor and PrPD across the disease progression as well as the increased GABA-like immunoreactivity in various brain regions of scrapie-infected hamsters starting from 21 dpi [62, 63]. The weak inhibitory activity of GABA(A) receptor may be associated with why seizure is common in prion disease.

Another way of studying the specific effects of exposure to toxic PrPD is through assessing the acute response of cells [5, 64]. A recent study has reported that acute exposure of *ex vivo* hippocampal slices to *ex vivo* mouse-adapted human prions (M1000 and MU02) disrupts CA1 LTP by causing dysfunctions of both pre- and postsynaptic activity [5]. With a similar approach, one study has reported that a 24-hour exposure of a mouse-adapted scrapie (RML) to cultured primary neuronal cells from wild type mice causes reduction of spontaneous neuronal activity due to a substantial loss of dendritic spines [23, 64]. The data show that, prior to developing clinical prion disease, neuronal cells modeling acquired prion disease have already undergone substantial biochemical and physiological changes.

3.2 Genetic prion diseases

Genetic prion diseases have been modeled in mice as well as in cultured cells. Genetic prion diseases are caused by disease-related mutations in the *prnp* gene. These diseases are autosomal dominant, therefore only one copy of the mutant allele is required to cause disease. Using these models, cellular and physiological changes can be measured during the asymptomatic stage prior to the onset of clinical signs, or before the misfolded PrPD becomes detectable [29, 65, 66]. Tg(PG14) mice, expressing a nine repeat insertion in the prion octapeptide region, display significant motor deficits prior to neuronal degeneration [65]. These early motor disturbances are associated with poor synaptic transmissions in cerebellar glutamatergic neurons due to a dysfunction in the mechanism that traffics and anchors voltage-gated calcium channels onto the cell membrane [65]. While the mechanisms of these abnormalities are likely due to a loss of functional PrPC or corruption of normal PrPC roles, the peptide insertion may directly yield PrPD species that are neurotoxic, resembling the pathophysiological mechanism of other diseases with repeat insertion such as Huntington's disease. Mouse models of familial CJD (Tg(CJD)) with the D178N mutation and a valine at codon 129, exhibit significant dysfunction of hippocampal CA1 LTP and metaplasticity during the presymptomatic stage (**Figure 1(4)**), which is approximately 50% of the disease progression, to the early onset of clinical disease [29, 66].

In cultured cells, expression of PrP P101L, a point mutant of mouse PrP that is equivalent to P102L mutation in GSS, significantly enhances inward currents and cell death despite a lack of insoluble PrPD (**Figure 1(5)**) [35, 36]. Similarly, cells expressing G113V or G130V mutations (models of genetic CJD and GSS) have minimal levels of insoluble PrPD but display increased inward currents [35]. Based on the role of PrPC as a regulator of ion channel activity (as described previously), the enhanced inward currents are likely due to a loss of PrPC functionality. However, exogenous PrP mutant lacking residues 105–125 while containing the membrane anchor motif can directly mediate membrane pore formation that increases sodium and calcium inward currents [67]. This finding suggests that the PrP mutant directly mediates neurotoxicity. Consistently, one study has revealed that the introduction of nanomolar concentrations of an exogenous PrP mutant lacking the residues 106–126 to rat forebrain neurons enhances the neuronal excitability by disrupting the whole-cell outward potassium currents, including the currents of calcium-activated potassium channels, which subsequently impairs the inhibitory activity of GABA [68]. This finding is consistent with Tg(CJD) mice exhibiting high susceptibility to kainite-induced seizure [65], and the report of carriers of the E200K mutation displaying increased MRI cortical hyperintensity during the early onset of clinical disease [1]. Taken together, PrPD species in genetic prion diseases appear to cause a significant dysfunction of inward and outward ion currents, which can disrupt the role of inhibitory neurons, thereby leading to enhanced neuronal excitability and consequently cell death.

4. Conclusions

PrPC plays a variety of essential roles in neuronal electrical signaling. PrPC maintains electrophysiological phenomena associated with cognition and behaviour by regulating ion channels activity, calcium homeostasis, inhibitory neuronal activity, various intracellular signal transduction pathways, and peripheral nerve myelination. These roles have been determined through two main experimental approaches including (1) knocking out of PrPC expression to completely abolish the roles of PrPC, and (2) deletion of specific PrP amino acid residues to change PrPC functions. Importantly, prior to the overt degeneration of neurons during the disease's progression, some of the disease-related neuronal dysfunctions are very similar to the altered neuro-physiological properties evident when PrPC is abolished or mutated. The reduction of LTP, impaired medium and late afterhyperpolarizations, disrupted calcium homeostasis, and weak inhibitory activity of GABA(A)R (**Figure 1**), are evident in mice devoid of PrPC as well as in mice and rats at the stages (asymptomatic to early onset) of prion diseases caused by exposure to infectious PrPD. In addition, the hyperactivity exhibited by neurons lacking the charged and hydrophobic residues of PrP is also evident in neurons of mice and cells harboring the disease-related mutants such as the D178N/129V and P101L (**Figure 1**). Further, some of the disease-related neuronal dysfunctions such as the reduction of LTP and spontaneous neuronal activity are evident in neuronal cells exposure to neurotoxic PrPD, which indicates that another way PrPC contributes to disease pathogenesis is by gaining a neurotoxic role. Overall, while the specific mechanisms of PrPC and PrPD engagement with the neuronal electrical signaling pathways remain to be elucidated, there are clear connections between the neurophysiological changes during diseases pathogenesis and the loss or corruption of PrPC function.

Acknowledgements

This research was supported by the Intramural Research Program of the NIH, Rocky Mountain Laboratories. We thank Austin J. Athman for his assistance in designing the figure.

Conflict of interest

Authors declare no "conflict of interest."

Abbreviations

AMPARs	α-amino-3-hydroxy-5-methyl-4-isoxazolepropionic acid receptors
CJD	Creutzfeldt-Jakob disease
EEG	electroencephalography
fMRI	functional magnetic resonance imaging
GABARs	gamma-aminobutyric acid receptors

GPI	glycosylphosphadiylinositol
GPI−/−	GPI anchorless
GSS	Gerstmann-Straussler-Scheinker syndrome
KR	kainate receptor
KCa	calcium-dependent potassium channel
LTD	long-term depression
LTP	long-term potentiation
MEG	magnetoencephalography
NMDARs	N-methyl-D-aspartate receptors
PrP	total prion protein species
PrPC	normal prion protein
PrPD	disease-causing PrP
RML	Rocky Mountain Laboratory prion
STP	short-term potentiation

Author details

Simote T. Foliaki, Bradley R. Groveman and Cathryn L. Haigh*
Division of Intramural Research, Laboratory of Persistent Viral Diseases, Rocky Mountain Laboratories, National Institute of Allergy and Infectious Diseases, National Institutes of Health, Hamilton, MT, USA

*Address all correspondence to: cathryn.haigh@nih.gov

References

[1] Kim MO et al. Genetic PrP prion diseases. Cold Spring Harbor Perspectives in Biology. 2018;**10**(5):pii:a033134

[2] Watts JC, Prusiner SB. Experimental models of inherited PrP prion diseases. Cold Spring Harbor Perspectives in Medicine. 2017;7(11):pii:a027151

[3] Brandner S, Jaunmuktane Z. Prion disease: Experimental models and reality. Acta Neuropathologica. 2017;**133**(2):197-222

[4] Nabavi S et al. Engineering a memory with LTD and LTP. Nature. 2014;**511**(7509):348-352

[5] Foliaki ST et al. Prion acute synaptotoxicity is largely driven by protease-resistant PrPSc species. PLoS Pathogens. 2018;**14**(8):e1007214

[6] Schulz PE. Long-term potentiation involves increases in the probability of neurotransmitter release. Proceedings of the National Academy of Sciences of the United States of America. 1997;**94**(11):5888-5893

[7] Luscher C, Malenka RC. NMDA receptor-dependent long-term potentiation and long-term depression (LTP/LTD). Cold Spring Harbor Perspectives in Biology. 2012;**4**(6):1-15

[8] Lee JS et al. Presynaptic release probability and readily releasable pool size are regulated by two independent mechanisms during posttetanic potentiation at the calyx of held synapse. The Journal of Neuroscience. 2008;**28**(32):7945-7953

[9] Wang L et al. Changes in potassium channel modulation may underlie afterhyperpolarization plasticity in oxytocin neurons during late pregnancy. Journal of Neurophysiology. 2018;**119**(5):1745-1752

[10] Powell AD et al. Alterations in Ca^{2+}–buffering in prion-null mice: Association with reduced afterhyperpolarizations in CA1 hippocampal neurons. The Journal of Neuroscience. 2008;**28**(15):3877-3886

[11] Liao D, Scannevin RH, Huganir R. Activation of silent synapses by rapid activity-dependent synaptic recruitment of AMPA receptors. The Journal of Neuroscience. 2001;**21**(16):6008-6017

[12] Wulf MA, Senatore A, Aguzzi A. The biological function of the cellular prion protein: An update. BMC Biology. 2017;**15**(1):34

[13] Herms J et al. Evidence of presynaptic location and function of the prion protein. The Journal of Neuroscience. 1999;**19**(20):8866-8875

[14] Khosravani H et al. Prion protein attenuates excitotoxicity by inhibiting NMDA receptors. The Journal of Cell Biology. 2008;**181**(3):551-565

[15] Um JW et al. Alzheimer amyloid-beta oligomer bound to postsynaptic prion protein activates Fyn to impair neurons. Nature Neuroscience. 2012;**15**(9):1227-1235

[16] Fournier JG et al. Ultrastructural localization of cellular prion protein (PrPc) in synaptic boutons of normal hamster hippocampus. Comptes Rendus de l'Académie des Sciences. Série III. 1995;**318**(3):339-344

[17] Laine J et al. Cellular and subcellular morphological localization of normal prion protein in rodent cerebellum. The European Journal of Neuroscience. 2001;**14**(1):47-56

[18] Moya KL et al. Immunolocalization of the cellular prion protein in normal brain. Microscopy Research and Technique. 2000;**50**(1):58-65

[19] Bailly Y et al. Prion protein (PrPc) immunocytochemistry and expression of the green fluorescent protein reporter gene under control of the bovine PrP gene promoter in the mouse brain. The Journal of Comparative Neurology. 2004;**473**(2):244-269

[20] Gohel C et al. Ultrastructural localization of cellular prion protein (PrPc) at the neuromuscular junction. Journal of Neuroscience Research. 1999;**55**(2):261-267

[21] Robinson SW et al. Prion protein facilitates synaptic vesicle release by enhancing release probability. Human Molecular Genetics. 2014;**23**(17):4581-4596

[22] Fuhrmann M et al. Loss of the cellular prion protein affects the Ca^{2+} homeostasis in hippocampal CA1 neurons. Journal of Neurochemistry. 2006;**98**(6):1876-1885

[23] Fang C et al. Prions activate a p38 MAPK synaptotoxic signaling pathway. PLoS Pathogens. 2018;**14**(9):e1007283

[24] Collinge J et al. Prion protein is necessary for normal synaptic function. Nature. 1994;**370**(6487):295-297

[25] Criado JR et al. Mice devoid of prion protein have cognitive deficits that are rescued by reconstitution of PrP in neurons. Neurobiology of Disease. 2005;**19**(1-2):255-265

[26] Curtis J et al. Age-dependent loss of PTP and LTP in the hippocampus of PrP-null mice. Neurobiology of Disease. 2003;**13**(1):55-62

[27] Schmitz M et al. Behavioral abnormalities in prion protein knockout mice and the potential relevance of PrP(C) for the cytoskeleton. Prion. 2014;**8**(6):381-386

[28] Lledo PM et al. Mice deficient for prion protein exhibit normal neuronal excitability and synaptic transmission in the hippocampus. Proceedings of the National Academy of Sciences of the United States of America. 1996;**93**(6):2403-2407

[29] Bertani I et al. Inhibition of IL-1beta signaling normalizes NMDA-dependent neurotransmission and reduces seizure susceptibility in a mouse model of Creutzfeldt-Jakob disease. The Journal of Neuroscience. 2017;**37**(43):10278-10289

[30] Bueler H et al. Normal development and behaviour of mice lacking the neuronal cell-surface PrP protein. Nature. 1992;**356**(6370):577-582

[31] Prestori F et al. Altered neuron excitability and synaptic plasticity in the cerebellar granular layer of juvenile prion protein knock-out mice with impaired motor control. The Journal of Neuroscience. 2008;**28**(28):7091-7103

[32] Fan J et al. Reduced hyperpolarization-activated current contributes to enhanced intrinsic excitability in cultured hippocampal neurons from PrP(−/−) mice. Frontiers in Cellular Neuroscience. 2016;**10**:74

[33] Mercer RC et al. The prion protein modulates A-type K+ currents mediated by Kv4.2 complexes through dipeptidyl aminopeptidase-like protein 6. The Journal of Biological Chemistry. 2013;**288**(52):37241-37255

[34] Solomon IH, Schepker JA, Harris DA. Prion neurotoxicity: Insights from prion protein mutants. Current Issues in Molecular Biology. 2010;**12**(2):51-61

[35] Solomon IH et al. An N-terminal polybasic domain and cell surface localization are required for mutant prion protein toxicity. The Journal of Biological Chemistry. 2011;**286**(16):14724-14736

[36] Solomon IH, Huettner JE, Harris DA. Neurotoxic mutants of the prion protein induce spontaneous ionic currents in cultured cells. The Journal of Biological Chemistry. 2010;**285**(34):26719-26726

[37] Li A et al. Neonatal lethality in transgenic mice expressing prion protein with a deletion of residues 105-125. The EMBO Journal. 2007;**26**(2):548-558

[38] Alvarez-Laviada A et al. The inhibition of functional expression of calcium channels by prion protein demonstrates competition with alpha2delta for GPI-anchoring pathways. The Biochemical Journal. 2014;**458**(2):365-374

[39] Mazzone GL, Nistri A. Modulation of extrasynaptic GABAergic receptor activity influences glutamate release and neuronal survival following excitotoxic damage to mouse spinal cord neurons. Neurochemistry International. 2019;**128**:175-185

[40] Rangel A et al. Regulation of GABA(a) and glutamate receptor expression, synaptic facilitation and long-term potentiation in the hippocampus of prion mutant mice. PLoS One. 2009;**4**(10):e7592

[41] Le Pichon CE et al. Olfactory behavior and physiology are disrupted in prion protein knockout mice. Nature Neuroscience. 2009;**12**(1):60-69

[42] Bremer J et al. Axonal prion protein is required for peripheral myelin maintenance. Nature Neuroscience. 2010;**13**(3):310-318

[43] Rial D et al. Cellular prion protein modulates age-related behavioral and neurochemical alterations in mice. Neuroscience. 2009;**164**(3):896-907

[44] Collins SJ, Lawson VA, Masters CL. Transmissible spongiform encephalopathies. The Lancet. 2004;**363**(9402):51-61

[45] Ferreira DG et al. Alpha-synuclein interacts with PrPC to induce cognitive impairment through mGluR5 and NMDAR2B. Nature Neuroscience. 2017;**20**(11):1569-1579

[46] Aguzzi A, Falsig J. Prion propagation, toxicity and degradation. Nature Neuroscience. 2012;**15**(7):936-939

[47] Zhang D et al. Targeting glutamatergic and cellular prion protein mechanisms of amyloid β-mediated persistent synaptic plasticity disruption: Longitudinal studies. Neuropharmacology. 2017;**121**:231-246

[48] Hu N-W et al. mGlu5 receptors and cellular prion protein mediate amyloid-β-facilitated synaptic long-term depression in vivo. Nature Communications. 2014;**5**(1):3374

[49] Cunningham C et al. Synaptic changes characterize early behavioural signs in the ME7 model of murine prion disease. The European Journal of Neuroscience. 2003;**17**(10):2147-2155

[50] Alibhai J et al. Distribution of misfolded prion protein seeding activity alone does not predict regions of neurodegeneration. PLoS Biology. 2016;**14**(11):e1002579

[51] Johnston AR et al. Synaptic plasticity in the CA1 area of the hippocampus of scrapie-infected mice. Neurobiology of Disease. 1998;**5**(3):188-195

[52] Fuhrmann M et al. Dendritic pathology in prion disease starts at the synaptic spine. The Journal of Neuroscience. 2007;**27**(23):6224-6233

[53] Barreca ML et al. Pharmacological agents targeting the cellular prion protein. Pathogens. 2018;**7**(1):pii:E27

[54] Weckhuysen D et al. Genetic Creutzfeldt-Jakob disease mimicking chronic inflammatory demyelinating polyneuropathy. Neurology Neuroimmunology & Neuroinflammation. 2015;**2**(6):e173

[55] Baiardi S et al. Prion-related peripheral neuropathy in sporadic Creutzfeldt-Jakob disease. Journal of Neurology, Neurosurgery, and Psychiatry. 2019;**90**(4):424-427

[56] Mallucci GR et al. Targeting cellular prion protein reverses early cognitive deficits and neurophysiological dysfunction in prion-infected mice. Neuron. 2007;**53**(3):325-335

[57] Pruisner SB. Novel proteinaceous infectious particles cause scrapie. Science. 1982;**216**:136-144

[58] Collinge J. Mammalian prions and their wider relevance in neurodegenerative diseases. Nature. 2016;**539**(7628):217-226

[59] Chiti Z et al. An integrated, temporal study of the behavioural, electrophysiological and neuropathological consequences of murine prion disease. Neurobiology of Disease. 2006;**22**(2):363-373

[60] Barrow PA et al. Intrinsic physiological and morphological properties of principal cells of the Hippocampus and Neocortex in hamsters infected with Scrapie. Neurobiology of Disease. 1999;**6**:406-423

[61] Trifilo MJ et al. Scrapie-induced defects in learning and memory of transgenic mice expressing anchorless prion protein are associated with alterations in the gamma aminobutyric acid-ergic pathway. Journal of Virology. 2008;**82**(20):9890-9899

[62] Lu P, Sturman JA, Bolton DC. Altered GABA distribution in hamster brain is an early molecular consequence of infection by scrapie prions. Brain Research. 1995;**681**(1-2):235-241

[63] Bouzamondo-Bernstein E et al. The neurodegeneration sequence in prion diseases: Evidence from functional, morphological and ultrastructural studies of the GABAergic system. Journal of Neuropathology and Experimental Neurology. 2004;**63**(8):882-899

[64] Fang C et al. A neuronal culture system to detect prion Synaptotoxicity. PLoS Pathogens. 2016;**12**(5):e1005623

[65] Senatore A et al. Mutant PrP suppresses glutamatergic neurotransmission in cerebellar granule neurons by impairing membrane delivery of VGCC alpha(2)delta-1 subunit. Neuron. 2012;**74**(2):300-313

[66] Dossena S et al. Mutant prion protein expression causes motor and memory deficits and abnormal sleep patterns in a transgenic mouse model. Neuron. 2008;**60**(4):598-609

[67] Chu NK et al. A C-terminal membrane anchor affects the interactions of prion proteins with lipid membranes. The Journal of Biological Chemistry. 2014;**289**(43):30144-30160

[68] Alier K et al. Ionic mechanisms of action of prion protein fragment PrP(106-126) in rat basal forebrain neurons. Journal of Neuroscience Research. 2010;**88**(10):2217-2227

Section 6

Neurodegenerative Processes in Epilepsy

Chapter 11

Molecular Mechanisms behind Initiation of Focal Seizure in Temporal Lobe Epilepsy: Computational Study

Ruchi Jakhmola Mani and Deepshikha Pande Katare

Abstract

Epilepsy is a noncommunicable disease of the brain that affects people of all ages. The chapter aims to identify protein targets and their mechanism of action behind temporal lobe epilepsy. Differentially expressed proteins in temporal lobe epilepsy (TLE) were used to derive a hypothesis demonstrating routes of protein interactions causing focal seizure and identification of putative target receptor for its treatment. Text mining was done by constructing a Boolean query with keywords such as temporal lobe epilepsy, focal seizures, proteomics, etc., in different scientific search engines. The proteins were further used for creating protein interaction network and analysed for their role in focal epileptic seizure pathway. The most appropriate route for initiation of seizure was observed to be route 3. It describes the dysregulated signal transduction from adenosine A1 receptor (ADORA1) to gamma-aminobutyric acid (GABA) B receptor 1 (GABBR1). This causes electrical imbalance and hyper-excitation of neurons that lead to focal seizure. The study also predicts that YWHAZ (3-monooxygenase/tryptophan 5-monooxygenase activation protein zeta) could be the potential target for preventing focal seizures. The network framed in this study is ideal for studying the cascades of events that may occur during focal seizures in TLE and is useful in drug discovery.

Keywords: temporal lobe epilepsy, focal seizures

1. What is epilepsy?

Epilepsy is the world's fourth most common neurological disorders. As indicated by the International League Against Epilepsy (ILAE), seizure is a transient of signs or appearances on the account of irregular, over the top, or synchronous neuronal development in the cerebrum. According to the WHO, 50 million people worldwide have epilepsy, and it is the fourth most common disease after Alzheimer's [1]. Epilepsy is an electrical unevenness in the cerebrum because of a few reasons like inactive way of life, hereditary distortions, hypoxic conditions, cranial harm, aggravation, or expansion in oxidative anxiety levels in the body, et cetera. A seizure is a sudden surge of electrical movement in the cerebrum. Seizures control how a man shows up or represents a brief span period. Neuronal cells either energize or repress (stop) other neuronal cells from sending messages. As a rule, there is an equalization of cells that energize and stop these messages. However, when a seizure occurs, there might be a lot of or too little action, bringing about an imbalance in the middle of exciting and halting movement. The nature of seizures varies, because the lobes of the brain control different behaviors, movements, and experiences. The accurate reason for a seizure is still obscure.

Some common causes of epilepsy are as follows:

- Low oxygen during birth
- Head injuries that occur during birth or due to accidents during youth or adulthood
- Brain tumors
- Genetic conditions that result in brain injury, such as tuberous sclerosis
- Infections such as meningitis or encephalitis

Because epilepsy is caused by abnormal activity in brain cells, seizures can affect any process your brain coordinates. Seizure signs and symptoms may include:

- Temporary confusion
- A staring spell
- Uncontrollable jerking movements of the arms and legs
- Loss of consciousness or awareness
- Psychic symptoms

Symptoms vary depending on the type of seizure. In most cases, a person with epilepsy will tend to have the same type of seizure each time, so the symptoms will be similar from episode to episode.

2. Focal seizures

Epilepsy comprises of more than 40 clinical disorders and is characterized by repeated seizures. Approximately 30% of patients treated with antiepileptic drugs (AEDs) are lacking control on seizures [2]. Seizure is a transient state of electrical imbalance in the brain. There are different types of seizures such as generalized, focal, and other types which hinder the normal functioning of the brain and cause epilepsy. Temporal lobe epilepsy is the most common seizure disorder in adults. The main cause for TLE is hippocampal sclerosis, and it constitutes around 80% of TLE cases [3]. The incidence rate of TLE was reported as 10.4 per 100, and its prevalence is 1.7 per 1000 people [4, 5]. TLE can be sporadic, ordinarily with a positive family history, or it can give clear familial repeat [6]. There is 70% of neuronal loss within the hippocampal region along with repeated focal seizures [7]. The regular clinical signs of focal seizures include gazing, absence of responsiveness, and mouth or hand automatisms. Focal seizure is mainly caused by the malfunction of ion channels. External stimuli like infection, tumors, and cranial injuries upregulate adenosine and increase the permeability of the blood-brain barrier which results in excessive influx of neurotransmitters into the hippocampal region. Lesser reuptake of these inhibitory neurotransmitters like gamma-aminobutyric acid (GABA) and glutamate by the receptors from the synaptic cleft causes neuroexcitation [8].

A recent study showed that GABA levels were found to be lower in diseased state than normal conditions. GABA system and receptor agonists have been used in the past for decreasing the effect of a seizure [9]. AEDs such as benzodiazepines (including clonazepam and clobazam) increase the frequency of opening of GABA receptors, and barbiturates (such as phenobarbitone) increase the time period for receptor opening. Thus, these drugs affect the release and movement of GABA [10]. Besides their positive effects on cognition ability and behavioral domain, AEDs have adverse effects on human health.

In this chapter we have hypothesized a protein-protein interaction network which proposes a possible mechanism underlying a focal seizure at a molecular level. Several proteins in this pathway were differentially regulated which initiates a cascade of events downstream that negatively regulates GABA [11]. The downregulation of GABA causes electrical imbalance in the brain and hence leads to focal seizure. Although drugs are available for treating TLE, prevention from its side effects is questionable; therefore, we have proposed new receptor for preventing seizures.

3. Building a hypothesis

3.1 Building a local protein database for network assessment

Text mining was done by constructing a Boolean query with keywords such as temporal lobe epilepsy, focal seizures, proteomics, differential expression, and human in different scientific search engines and databases like PubMed Central, ScienceDirect, and Google Scholar. Several combinations of keywords were used to fetch research articles according to the study. Many research articles were obtained and screened manually for differentially expressed proteins in TLE. The proteins were further used to create protein-interaction network.

3.2 Creation of protein interaction network

Protein accession numbers were submitted to Cytoscape v2.6 software as query, and it gave a master network between the query proteins. The master network comprised of query proteins and their interacting partners. This network was created by BioGRID, IntAct, and other protein-protein interaction databases included in the Cytoscape framework. This network was accompanied with the most followed pathways ranked according to their e-values. E-value is an indicator that the results are independent of the protein queries chosen and the master network is unbiased i.e. the network is based on experimentally verified protein-protein interactions and hence are reflected in the network.

3.3 Framing and analysis of hypothesis

The master network was studied, and the proteins exclusively responsible for a focal seizure were extracted and linked to formulate a pathway that might be responsible for causing seizure in an epileptic brain. This hypothesis was formulated in a stepwise manner, and it explains the series of interactions that might occur in the brain during the initiation of a focal seizure in TLE.

4. Results

Proteins involved in TLE were collected after extensive literature survey. The network is in the form of ball and sticks. Balls represent protein nodes, and sticks represent the interaction between them. The proteins immediately next to the query proteins are called as first neighbors. These first neighbors are later connected to second neighbors and so on (**Figure 1**). The extensive networking between these proteins indicates their involvement in similar pathways or processes.

A total of 668 neighbor proteins were retrieved for query proteins. They were colored in white and gray balls. White balls represent the proteins following the similar pathways as do the query proteins, whereas the gray balls represent the proteins following dissimilar different pathways. The query and neighbor proteins were observed to be following NGF, NT, adhesion, MAPK, and few more pathways.

We have hypothesized a network of proteins which is suggested to be the mechanism behind seizures (**Figure 2**). The interactions were later segregated into smaller routes to understand the flow of information inside the brain during a seizure (**Figure 3(a)–(d)**). The starting point for the current study of routes was finalized to be adenosine A1 receptor (ADORA1), while the last (effector molecule) was chosen to be gamma-aminobutyric acid B receptor 1 (GABBR1), we have limited our hypothesis between these two proteins.

4.1 Route 1

Adenosine is observed to be upregulated in TLE. Later it binds with ADORA1 and inhibits the signal transducer activity of GNAS (guanine nucleotide-binding protein G(s) subunit alpha isoforms XLas) protein [12]. Further, GNAS which stimulates the activity of adenylate cyclase type 5 (ADCY5) when inhibited leads to inhibition of ADCY5, and as a result there is no production of secondary messenger cAMP (**Figure 3(a)**) [13]. ADCY5 is also regulated by protein kinase C alpha type (PRKCA), and it inhibits its catalytic activity. YWHAZ then acts as an adaptor

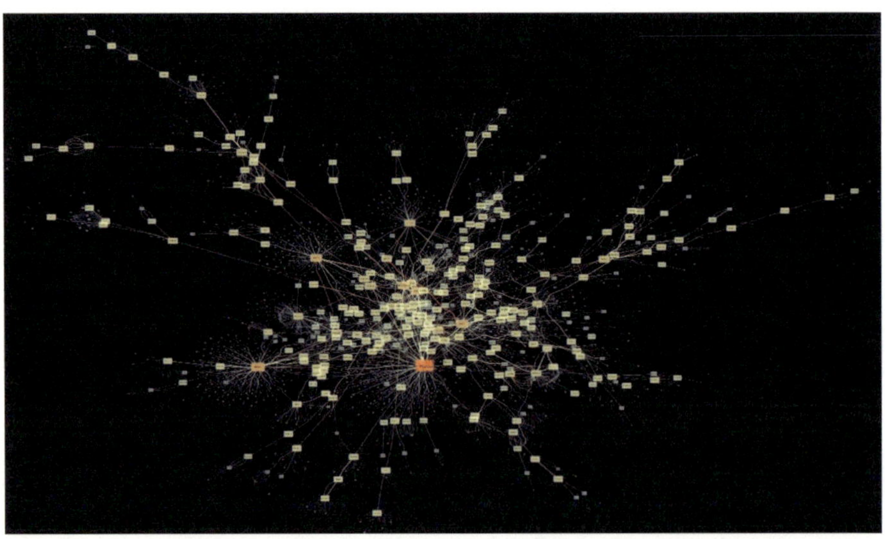

Figure 1.
The network generated by Cytoscapev2.7.2. The figure represents the master network, i.e., clusters of proteins communicating with each other during TLE conditions. It also reports the pathways mostly followed by the proteins involved in this network.

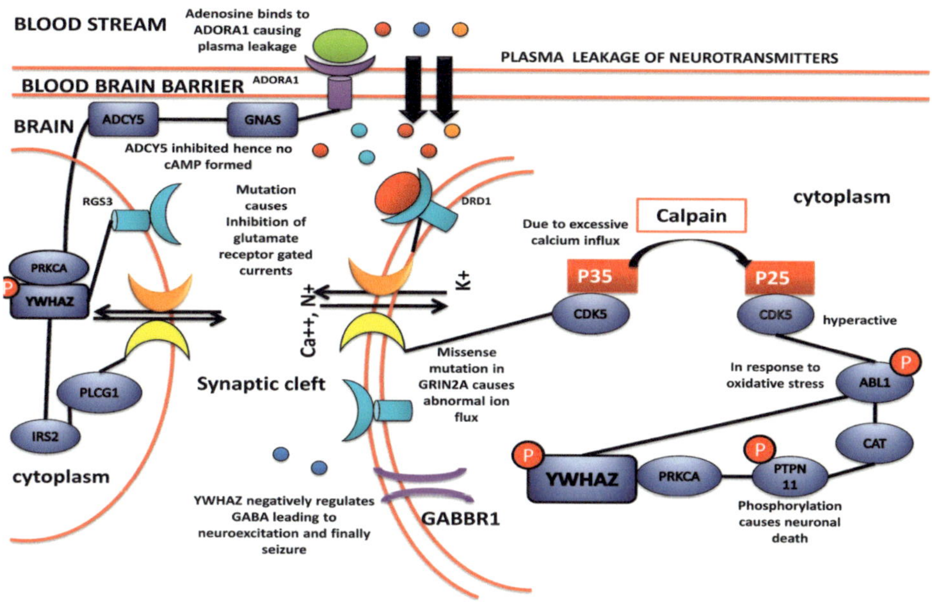

Figure 2.
Pictorial representation of seizure events in the brain during generalized seizures. The figure shows the detailed graphic representation of events occurring in the brain during focal seizure. Proteins involved in the hypothesis are shown in blue color. The process is redrawn as a simplified diagram for easy understanding.

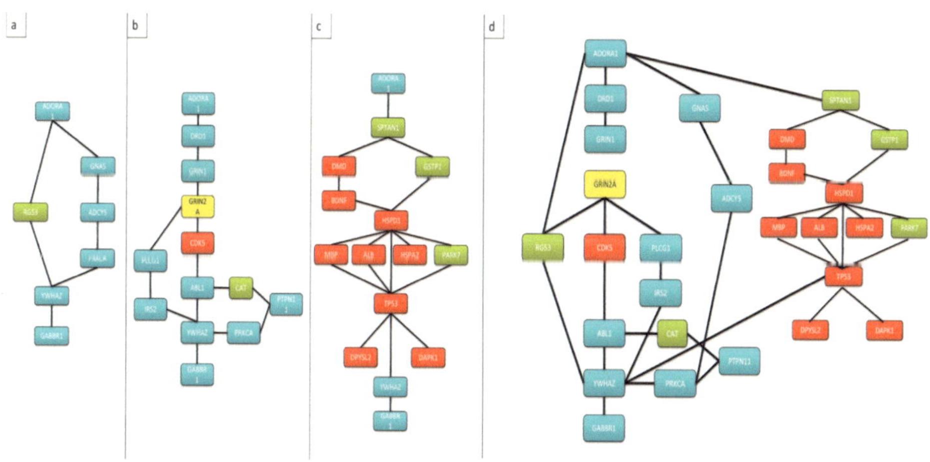

Figure 3.
The possible routes involved in a seizure: (a) route 1, (b) route 2, (c) route 3, and (d) simplified diagram of cumulative routes. The figure represents the different hypotheses of focal seizure generation via three different routes.

protein which interacts with PRKCA signaling molecule [14]. Ultimately YWHAZ negatively regulates GABA causing neuroexcitation, and hence seizure occurs [15].

Alternatively, ADORA1 is also inversely proportional to regulators of G protein signaling 3 (RGS3) which are G protein signaling molecules. RGS3 is downregulated by YWHAZ, causing no activation of MAP kinases which leads to altered cell growth and proliferation [16].

4.2 Route 2

Upregulation of adenosine in the body results in increased permeability of the BBB which leads to excessive influx of neurotransmitters [7]. Due to lesser reuptake of these neurotransmitters by DRD1(dopamine receptor D1), it inhibits the activity of ADCY5 leading to decreased production of cAMP(secondary messenger) [17]. Coupling of DRD1 and glutamate receptor, ionotropic, N-methyl, D-aspartate 1 (GRIN1) causes inhibition of NMDA glutamate receptor-gated currents. GRIN 1 and glutamate receptor, ionotropic, N-methyl, D-aspartate 2A (GRIN 2A) are subunits of NMDA receptor [18]. Missense mutation in GRIN2A initiates phospholipase c, gamma 1 (PLCG1) [19]. Initiation of PLCG1 separates phosphatidylinositol 4, 5-bisphosphate (PIP2) into the second messengers, diacylglycerol (DAG) and inositol 1, 4, 5-trisphosphate (IP3), which play a vital role in intracellular signal transduction. An interruption in this signaling pathway causes altered synaptic transmission (**Figure 3(b)**) [19]. When mutated GRIN2A interacts with PLCG1, it causes hindrance in the production of secondary messengers and ultimately alters the intracellular signal transduction. Thereafter, PLCG1 does not activate, and no phosphorylation of tyrosine kinases takes place. It further causes no stimulation of insulin receptor substrate 2 (IRS2) [20]. This results in negative regulation of insulin which is facilitated by association of IRS2 and YWHAZ. Then, YWHAZ ultimately downregulates GABA, causing a seizure.

Alternatively, it is known that GRIN1 is also responsible for verbal memory and its inhibition causes speech impairment during a seizure (**Figure 3(b)**). GRIN2A is significant for neuronal activity and development. But a missense mutation of GRIN2A leads to abnormal neuronal ion flux and electrical transmission leading to developmental abnormalities [21]. GRIN1 and GRIN2A are the two subunits of NMDA glutamate receptor. Mutated GRIN2A causes excessive Ca^{2+} influx which causes conversion of P35 to P25 by calcium-dependent protease, calpain, during neurotoxicity and contributes to the pathological state. Elevation in levels of P25 leads to hyperactivation of cyclin-dependent kinase 5 (CDK5) which causes impairment in behavior, cognition, and synaptic plasticity [22]. Further elevated levels of CDK5 and oxidative stress phosphorylates ABL proto-oncogene 1, non-receptor tyrosine kinase (ABL-1) which is a ubiquitous non-receptor tyrosine kinase which promotes apoptosis and cytoskeleton remodeling [23]. ABL-1 in response to oxidative stress downregulates catalase (CAT) activity [24]. CAT binds actively to tyrosine-protein phosphatase non-receptor 11 (PTPN11) which is responsible for RAS/MAPK signaling which further leads to apoptosis. Low levels of CAT cause decreased resistance of PTPN11 toward hydrogen peroxide [25]. PTPN11 is phosphorylated by PRKCA, triggering neuronal death. YWHAZ acts as an adaptor protein which interacts with PRKCA signaling molecule. In response to DNA damage, ABL-1 is targeted into the nucleus, and it phosphorylates YWHAZ causing the activation of JNK signaling which is responsible for apoptosis [26].

4.3 Route 3

ADORA1 is activated by the upregulation of adenosine due to any external stimulus [27]. As a result, the permeability of BBB increases causing influx of calcium ions. Further, activation of ADORA1 causes downregulation of spectrin alpha chain, non-erythrocytic 1 (SPTAN1) which regulates the entry of calcium ions in neurons [27]. Due to decreased availability of calcium ions, DMD (dystrophin) is upregulated, and no proper synaptic transmission takes place [28]. Simultaneously, SPTAN1 interacts with glutathione S-transferase P (GSTP1) which is an antioxidant enzyme, regulating CDK5; downregulation of GSTP1 causes downregulation of CDK5; hence neurodegeneration initiates. On the other hand, DMD interacts with brain-derived neurotrophic factor (BDNF) which controls the neuronal excitability, is upregulated, and causes hyperexcitability [29]. BDNF and GSTP1 together interact with HSPD1 (60 kDa heat shock protein, mitochondrial), which prevents misfolding of proteins, but it gets upregulated [30]. HSPD1 binds to five more proteins, namely, myelin basic protein (MBP), serum albumin (ALB), heat shock-related 70 kDa protein 2 (HSPA2), protein deglycase DJ-1 (PARK7), and cellular tumor antigen p53 (TP53). MBP forms the myelin sheath of a neuron, and its upregulation causes dysfunctioning of protein. The upregulation of ALB hinders its binding to the calcium ions which are leaked from the BBB and alter the osmotic pressure of neuronal cells [31]. Further HSPA2, which prevents aggregation of proteins, gets upregulated, it does not perform its function properly. PARK7 in response to increased oxidative stress does not perform its function of reducing the number of free radicals. The upregulation of TP53, a tumor suppressor protein, results in downregulation of apoptosis regulator Bcl-2 (BCL-2). BCL-2 induces apoptosis and causes neurodegeneration [32]. Further, TP53 interacts with YWHAZ which in response to oxidative stress arrests the cell cycle [33]. TP53 also interacts with dihydropyrimidinase-related protein 2 (DPYSL2) and death-associated protein kinase 1 (DAPK1). DPYSL2 modulates the growth of neurons which is upregulated and causes hindrance in transmission of electric signals, causing focal seizures. Normally, DAPK1 prevents autophagy in normal conditions, when the cell is under stress, it is elevated and causes destruction of neuronal cells [34].

From the abovementioned theories, the nearest and most realistic route for causing seizure generation is proposed to be route 3. This pathway was picked because it has those proteins which are differentially regulated and cause electrical irregularity in the brain, bringing on a focal seizure. Repetitive seizures cause weaknesses in cognizance, learning, and memory. Also, it has been seen the GABA levels were found to be low in brain tissue of epileptic patients. Real occasions during focal seizure are transformation of GRIN2A which brings about hindrance in neuronal particle flux. Our study concludes that the extended protein signal finally reaches to YWHAZ which causes hyperexcitation. This was due to inefficient binding of GABA to GABBR1 receptor (**Figure 2**).

5. Conclusion

The study hypothesized the series of protein-protein interactions which may potentially occur during a focal seizure. Out of the three plausible paths for the initiation of focal seizure, the most appropriate is route 3 which starts with upregulation of adenosine. Route 3 causes cell cycle arrest and starts the apoptosis of neuronal cells along with the hindrance in synaptic transmission [35].

Although AEDs have been formulated for numerous receptors, its generation is still an unresolved question. A study by Steinlein et al. showed that mutations in genes encoding for voltage-gated and ligand-gated ion channels like GABBR1 receptors and nicotinic acetylcholine receptors are mutated. These mutated receptors cause electrical imbalance in the brain [36].

Similarly, a study by Suls et al. suggested that some proteins undergo genetic mutations in TLE [37]. In the past research, it has been seen that mutations in GLUT1 causes epilepsy. GLUT1 is the major receptor for gluten molecule. GLUT1 mutation imbalances the concentration of gluten, K^+, and albumin across the BBB and impairs the K^+ buffering in the brain. Gluten metabolism and transport is also disturbed which becomes the major reason for neuronal excitability [38]. Some studies also suggested that seizure is caused due to mutation in CDK5 [39]. The modulation of GABAergic inhibition by NMDA receptors may cause the synaptic plasticity [40].

On the other hand, excessive influx of calcium ions leads to hindered synaptic transmission [35], due to which heat shock proteins are unable to perform their normal function. In response to oxidative stress proteins like BDNF, MBP, ALB, and TP53, DPYSL2 gets upregulated and induces apoptosis, hence causing neurodegeneration [22]. Then, YWHAZ finally binds to GABBR1 (helps in preventing ion leakage on the membrane and neuronal hyperactivity) and makes it unable to bind to GABA, which is an inhibitory neurotransmitter. Therefore, YWHAZ can be studied in future as a drug target for epileptic focal seizures.

To date, there were just a couple of protein receptors targeted for antiepileptic drugs which manage the pathology. Also, there are no medications to prevent a seizure, and no such receptor has been predicted for the same. Therefore, the present study proposes that the proteins involved in route 3 may give some understanding into the fundamental mechanism behind seizures. Protein that can be focused for designing AEDs can be YWHAZ.

Acknowledgements

We would like to acknowledge Dr. Ashok K. Chauhan, Founder President, Amity University Uttar Pradesh, Noida, for providing the infrastructure and support.

Author details

Ruchi Jakhmola Mani and Deepshikha Pande Katare*
Proteomics and Translational Research Lab, Centre for Medical Biotechnology, Amity Institute of Biotechnology, Amity University, Noida, India

*Address all correspondence to: dpkatare@amity.edu

References

[1] Banerjee PN, Filippi D, Hauser WA. The descriptive epidemiology of epilepsy—A review. Epilepsy Research. 2009;**85**:31-45

[2] Schiffer RB, Babigian HM. Behavioral disorders in multiple sclerosis, temporal lobe epilepsy, and amyotrophic lateral sclerosis: An epidemiologic study. Archives of Neurology. 1984;**41**:1067-1069

[3] Haneef Z, Lenartowicz A, Yeh HJ, et al. Functional connectivity of hippocampal networks in temporal lobe epilepsy. Epilepsia. 2014;**55**:137-145

[4] Clancy MJ, Clarke MC, Connor DJ, et al. The prevalence of psychosis in epilepsy; a systematic review and meta-analysis. BMC Psychiatry. 2014;**14**:1

[5] Rigau V, Morin M, Rousset MC, et al. Angiogenesis is associated with blood–brain barrier permeability in temporal lobe epilepsy. Brain. 2007;**130**:1942-1956

[6] Bedner P et al. Astrocyte uncoupling as a cause of human temporal lobe epilepsy. Brain. 2015;**138**(5):1208-1222

[7] Lapointe E, Deacon C, Bocti C, et al. Temporal lobe atrophy: Frequent in elderly with epilepsy of unknown etiology. Clinical Neurophysiology. 2016;**127**:e161

[8] Ben-Ari Y, Khalilov I, Kahle KT, et al. The GABA excitatory/inhibitory shift in brain maturation and neurological disorders. The Neuroscientist. 2012;**18**:467-486

[9] Briggs SW, Galanopoulou AS. Altered GABA signaling in early life epilepsies. Neural Plasticity. 2011;**2011**. Article ID 527605

[10] Jacob TC, Moss SJ, Jurd R. GABAA receptor trafficking and its role in the dynamic modulation of neuronal inhibition. Nature Reviews. Neuroscience. 2008;**9**:331-343

[11] Sebba J, Hogg LLJ. Profound Retardation and Multiple Impairment: Volume 3: Medical and Physical Care and Management. Springer; 1 Dec 2013

[12] Baraldi PG, Tabrizi MA, Fruttarolo F, et al. Recent improvements in the development of A2B adenosine receptor agonists. Purinergic Signal. 2008;**4**:287-303

[13] Hampton M, Melvin RG, Andrews MT. Transcriptomic analysis of brown adipose tissue across the physiological extremes of natural hibernation. PLOS One. 2013;**8**:e85157

[14] Gannon-Murakami L, Murakami K. Selective association of protein kinase C with 14-3-3 ζ in neuronally differentiated PC12 cells stimulatory and inhibitory effect of 14-3-3 ζ in vivo. The Journal of Biological Chemistry. 2002;**277**:23116-23122

[15] Couve A, Kittler JT, Uren JM, et al. Association of GABA B receptors and members of the 14-3-3 family of signaling proteins. Molecular and Cellular Neurosciences. 2001;**17**:317-328

[16] Kleppe R, Rosati S, Jorge-Finnigan A, et al. Phosphorylation dependence and stoichiometry of the complex formed by tyrosine hydroxylase and 14-3-3γ. Molecular & Cellular Proteomics. 2014;**13**:2017-2030

[17] Levy F, de Leon J. Dopamine ADHD/OCD theories: Is glutamine part of the story? Neurotransmitter. 2015;**2**

[18] Petralia RS, Al-Hallaq RA, Wenthold RJ. Trafficking and targeting

of NMDA receptors. Biology of the NMDA Receptor. 2009;**1**:149-200

[19] Jang HJ, Yang YR, Kim JK, et al. Phospholipase C-γ1 involved in brain disorders. Advances in Biological Regulation. 2013;**53**:51-62

[20] Ghorbani S, Fossbakk A, Jorge-Finnigan A, et al. Regulation of tyrosine hydroxylase is preserved across different homo-and heterodimeric 14-3-3 proteins. Amino Acids. 2016;**48**:1221-1229

[21] Clasadonte J, Dong J, Hines DJ, et al. Astrocyte control of synaptic NMDA receptors contributes to the progressive development of temporal lobe epilepsy. Proceedings of the National Academy of Sciences. 2013;**110**:17540-17545

[22] Hawasli AH, Bibb JA. Alternative roles for Cdk5 in learning and synaptic plasticity. Biotechnology Journal. 2007;**2**:941-948

[23] Chen L, Wang Z, Tang B, et al. Altered expression of c-Abl in patients with epilepsy and in a rat model. Synapse. 2014;**68**:306-316

[24] Cao C, Leng Y, Kufe D. Catalase activity is regulated by c-Abl and Arg in the oxidative stress response. The Journal of Biological Chemistry. 2003;**278**:29667-29675

[25] Yano S, Arroyo N, Yano N. SHP2 binds catalase and acquires a hydrogen peroxide-resistant phosphatase activity via integrin-signaling. FEBS Letters. 2004;**577**:327-332

[26] Yoshida K, Yamaguchi T, Natsume T, et al. JNK phosphorylation of 14-3-3 proteins regulates nuclear targeting of c-Abl in the apoptotic response to DNA damage. Nature Cell Biology. 2005;**7**:278-285

[27] da Silva Fernandes MJ, Amorim RP, Carneiro JE, et al. Proteomics-based strategy to identify biomarkers and pharmacological targets in temporal lobe epilepsy. In: Pharmacoresistance in Epilepsy. New York: Springer; 2013. pp. 115-126

[28] Lee TS, Eid T, Mane S, et al. Aquaporin-4 is increased in the sclerotic hippocampus in human temporal lobe epilepsy. Acta Neuropathologica. 2004;**108**:493-502

[29] Sadakata T, Shinoda Y, Oka M, et al. Reduced axonal localization of a Caps2 splice variant impairs axonal release of BDNF and causes autistic-like behavior in mice. Proceedings of the National Academy of Sciences. 2012;**109**:21104-21109

[30] Gammazza AM, Colangeli R, Orban G, et al. Hsp60 response in experimental and human temporal lobe epilepsy. Scientific Reports. 2015;**5**

[31] Van Vliet EA, da Costa AS, Redeker S, et al. Blood–brain barrier leakage may lead to progression of temporal lobe epilepsy. Brain. 2007;**130**:521-534

[32] Kilany A, Raouf ER, Gaber AA, et al. Elevated serum Bcl-2 in children with temporal lobe epilepsy. Seizure. 2012;**21**:250-253

[33] Waterman MJ, Stavridi ES, Waterman JL, et al. ATM-dependent activation of p53 involves dephosphorylation and association with 14-3-3 proteins. Nature Genetics. 1998;**19**:175-178

[34] Hainsworth AH, Allsopp RC, Jim A, et al. Death-associated protein kinase (DAPK1) in cerebral cortex of late-onset Alzheimer's disease patients and aged controls. Neuropathology and Applied Neurobiology. 2010;**36**:17-24

[35] Voss LJ, Jacobson G, Sleigh JW. Bridging the Gap—Understanding the Role of Gap Junctions in Seizures. IntechOpen Access Publisher; 2011

[36] White HS, Smith MD, Wilcox KS. Mechanisms of action of antiepileptic drugs. International Review of Neurobiology. 2007;**81**:85-110

[37] Scheffer IE, Berkovic SF. The genetics of human epilepsy. Trends in Pharmacological Sciences. 2003;**24**:428-433

[38] Suls A, Mullen SA, Weber YG, et al. Early-onset absence epilepsy caused by mutations in the glucose transporter GLUT1. Annals of Neurology. 2009;**66**:415-419

[39] Castrén M, Gaily E, Tengström C, et al. Epilepsy caused by CDKL5 mutations. European Journal of Paediatric Neurology. 2011;**15**(1):65-69

[40] Stelzer A, Slater NT, Bruggencate GT. Activation of NMDA receptors blocks GABAergic inhibition in an in vitro model of epilepsy. Nature. 1987;**326**(6114):698-701